Acknowledgements

This book is dedicated to my children Alex and Ariana and all the wonderful people who have helped with my research, a massive thank you to you all.

D0268953

Introduction

What is this book about?

Everything you see around you is there because someone thought about it, and then brought it to life, so it makes profound sense to say that you can create a perfect body of your choice by the power of your thoughts.

A majority of people think and believe that losing weight and maintaining it is all about eating healthy and exercising, forgetting that real health stems from the mind because the mind controls everything from the food choices you make to whether you keep active or not. The truth is that the mind has total control over the body, an example of this is you think and fantasize about having that fast food take away – then you proceed to buy it to the point of eating it, you see you have acted upon what your mind suggested, which all started as a thought. In other words your mind has controlled and decided on the choice of food you've made and this goes on to show you that your mind controls your choices and what goes into your body whether good or bad! And this is where all the hard work and changes have to begin. IN YOUR MIND.

The mind is a powerful tool in holding the power to the way we think, feel, act and behave, therefore its only fair to say that the mind dictates our life choices for instance what we chose to eat and whether we stay active or not. Therefore any attempts to any change of behavioural patterns and attitudes should also start in the mind, with a " thought" then "action" will follow. It's a fact that your body is a reflection of your thoughts, feelings,

5

attitudes and beliefs. And its also the power of the mind that holds the key for fast weight loss and maintaining it hence any weight loss starts in the mind! Therefore by learning to access and use the power of the mind through self-hypnosis, visualization, meditation, positive thinking and relaxation technique you can change any negative bad habits, thoughts, beliefs to change your body.

Programming your mind is crucial for healthy food choices, keeping and staying active, weight loss and maintenance , but it's only the starting point, once you've got the right mind-set then its time to look into your diet, remember "whatever goes into your body strengthens it or weakens it and "you are what you eat", so it's very important that you eat the right foods in the right amounts. In other words a balanced diet with proteins, carbohydrates, fats, vitamins and minerals and plenty of water. Be aware that if you eat more food than your body needs for daily functioning, activity and cell maintenance, you will put on weight.

Regardless, to lose weight and be able to manage it you need to lose the amount of calories that you eat and also increase your levels of exercise. The power of your mind will enable you to exercise and burn calories, build muscles, keep you fit and energetic, increase metabolism and reduce your risk of major illnesses such as heart disease, stroke, diabetes and some cancers by 50% and lower your risk of early death by up to 30%. Exercise is healthy for both body and mind whether it is walking, running, swimming, cycling, or playing sports it should be enjoyable and fun.

In summary, more and more people are giving up diets more than ever before, they have come to a conclusion that diets don't work as more often people pile the weight back on after the dieting period. The truth lies behind the power of your mind and how to use that power to your advantage analysing what you eat and your activity levels. These are the only easy and proven ways to stay healthy, lose weight and manage it.

Benefits of this book
- o By reading this book you will learn how to access and use the power of the mind not only to make healthy choices but also to lose weight and maintain it. When you access the power of your mind, you access well being. By using self-hypnosis, visualization, meditation, positive thinking, positive statements and relaxation techniques.
- o In this book you learn about healthy eating and its benefits, illnesses associated with un-healthy diets, losing weight, and maintaining a healthy weight.
- o Furthermore in this book you will learn about exercising to stay healthy, lose weight and maintain the weight loss and also discover various exercises and their benefits to a healthy body and mind.
- o And last but not least this book goes on to show you how self-motivation can help you to initiate the decision to make changes, help you to push through the challenges and achieve your goals be it losing weight, exercise daily or maintain your ideal weight.

Why write this book?

My reason for writing this book is very simple, it's to show you how to stay healthy, lose weight and also be able to maintain it in a very easy, instinctive and natural way by accessing and working with your mind in a positive way, eating the right foods and exercising without having to spend your money, time and energy on diets and addictive toxic diet pills with plenty of side effects which don't work anyway!

It has come to my attention that a vast majority of books on the market about healthy eating and losing weight are aimed at drawing reading audiences towards writers' practices or surgeries, however this book is primarily focussing on giving you the power to help yourself, There is nothing more empowering and rewarding than taking control, you know why you are in this situation and its you who has the power to get you out of the situation, no one else. So take charge NOW.

I hope that you benefit from reading this book, find it informative and that it inspires you to achieve your goal. Remember that the power is in your hands to act now, trust that inner strength within you to carry you on to fulfil your utmost dreams and desires.

Thank you.

Josephine Spire

****

Mind Power and Healthy Eating: The Art of Losing Weight and
Staying Healthy

Table of Contents

****

Mind Power and Healthy Eating: The Art of Losing Weight and Staying Healthy

Part One

MIND POWER TECHNIQUES

The mind is that element of a human being that facilitates and enables thoughts, feelings and experiences. The human mind consists of two parts: the conscious mind and the subconscious mind.

The Conscious Mind: is the part of the mind that is responsible for logic, reasoning, accepting or rejecting information and it's also responsible for decision making.

The Subconscious Mind: is the part of the mind that stores information, it functions at a much deeper level than the conscious mind and it's not limited by logic or reasoning.

The mind is a powerful tool and it's true that any weight loss starts in the mind with a thought, then action follows. And it's a fact that your body is a reflection of your thoughts, feelings, attitudes and beliefs. And it's also the power of the mind that holds the key to healthy eating, weight loss and maintenance of weight loss. Therefore by learning to access and use the power of the mind through self-hypnosis, visualization, positive thinking-affirmations, meditation, and relaxation techniques, you can change any bad or negative habits, thoughts, attitudes or beliefs to finally change the way you look.

The body and mind are connected in a way that your body will respond to the way you think, feel and behave around food. It's well known that your body is a reflection of what goes on in the mind, so learning to control your eating habits and body weight will be your strongest tools to keep healthy and achieve your perfect weight. The only proven way to lose weight is by eating healthily and keeping active but by changing the way you think and act will tremendously speed up your weight loss plan. It's your mind that holds the power to fast weight loss and keeping you on track. Rest assured that mind power and action will get you your desired goal by programming your mind through:

- o Self-Hypnosis
- o Visualization
- o Positive thinking
- o Positive statements
- o Meditation
- o Relaxation techniques

A healthy mind versus an unhealthy mind

A healthy mind	Unhealthy mind
- Healthy diet	- Poor diet
- Exercise	- Lack of exercise
- Positive thinking	- Negative thinking
- Hypnosis	- Excessive stress
- Meditation	- Alcohol, smoking

- Relaxation techniques

- Hydration

- Healthy restful sleep pattern

- Deep breathing

- Outdoors

- Drug abuse

- Dehydration

-Lack of sleep

-Shallow breathing

-Excessive TV
gaming,
computers,
mobile phones

Change

Before we go further to explore the mind techniques and how they can help you change and enhance your life in the way you want it to, I would like to say a few important words about change. Lets face it you are reading this book because you want to change your behaviours, attitudes, beliefs or thoughts that are holding you back. First you don't have to wait until the new year to make resolutions for change, new years resolutions fail to work for people and are often broken because people try to make changes based on a specific date rather than making changes because they are ready for them and want them to take place. Some people try to change for all the wrong reasons, for instance because they are doing it to please someone or having been pushed to change, moreover it is very unlikely to yield any success if you're changing for other people, the desire and drive has to come from within yourself for change to take full positive effect. In other words if you want to lose weight because you want to please someone then you're coming at this from the wrong angle. It's a good thing to please other people especially the ones you love and care for but you have to please yourself first, lose weight for yourself because of all the healthy benefits this has for you. By putting yourself first and making yourself happy you will make your loved ones happy too because you're happy, healthy, fit and look great. And because the desire comes from within yourself your motivation and rate of success is guaranteed to be very high.

Second, you have to want to change and you have to believe in yourself and your abilities to achieve whatever you're aiming to achieve, if you do that failure will never be an option. If you don't make that decision to change, you will forever be stuck in your own prison and you won't learn new things. Accept and embrace change, it will make you stronger and open new doors for you. We all struggle in life but you have to make things happen in your life and try as much as you can not to give up, otherwise you will never know how close you were to succeeding!

Third, never make assumptions before even trying, yes change is going to be hard and testing but with determination you will triumph, assumption is always unproductive, damaging and the lowest form of knowledge you will ever come across. So don't assume that you can't do it because you can, don't ever let other people judge you and discourage you, it doesn't matter what you look like, where you come from, your age, disability or whatever it is. Whatever makes you different from anyone else is your uniqueness, you are not meant to look like everyone else. In my understanding no one human being should ever be written off, I believe that given a chance every single one of us can shine and succeed as we are all here to serve a purpose and to solve a problem for one another, for example a doctor is here to heal people, a farmer grows crops and rears animals to feed people, a mechanic looks after your car, the person who works on the till at the supermarket does a tremendous job too, it doesn't matter what job you do however small or less important you think it is, you're special and you change people's lives everyday.

To make those changes in your life, you have to work with your subconscious mind, as the quality of your thoughts will affect and shape the quality of your life. To make those changes you have to consider;

o What your dreams are as dreams are built on desire and desire pushes you to achieve those dreams.
o What are you getting from your achievements-the benefits.
o Make that decision to change
o Make your decision into a reality

Change is like the earth's seasons, it's endless. We have to align with nature and learn from it as from nature we can truly learn about change and embrace it. Change can be testing, painful, exciting, very slow, fast, rewarding and continuous. Change is constant and part of life, change triggers development and has numerous rewards and can yield immense success.

**

MIND POWER TECHNIQUES

Self-Hypnosis

Self-hypnosis is a simple way of training your mind how to relax so that you can gain access to the subconscious mind and be able to introduce new positive suggestions, statements or affirmations to help you eliminate , improve and overcome blocks, negative thinking, self defeating beliefs and doubts and also create positive changes in your life. For self-hypnosis to be effective, you have to deeply relax and reach a heightened level of concentration and relaxation for the positive suggestions to be implanted into your subconscious mind. In a very deep relaxed state your conscious mind goes to rest or steps aside to give way to your subconscious mind which is responsible for storing everything that you have ever experienced in life, for example feelings, images, sounds, tastes, and smells. When under hypnosis all your senses will remain fully alert throughout the whole process. This is because hypnosis is a natural, relaxed state of mind that you can choose to enter anytime you want, as a matter of fact you enter hypnosis everyday without even noticing that you're doing it!

Like any other new skill, you will have to practice self-hypnosis as many times as you can to be able to fully train your mind how to relax and before you know it, you will be reaping the benefits! Hypnosis is;

- o A natural state of mind
- o You're in control
- o You're aware of all your senses and fully alert

- o Harmless
- o You can come out of it any time you wish to

Hypnosis is not;

- o Mind manipulation or tricking
- o Weird
- o Mind control
- o Unconsciousness
- o Deep sleep

However, self-hypnosis should not be used by people who suffer from psychosis or other types of personality disorders, are using any form of drugs or alcohol.

How does Self-Hypnosis work ?

As well as helping you to maintain good health and lose weight, self-hypnosis can be applied to many areas of your life as you obtain the ability to talk to your subconscious and there are many benefits to be achieved from practicing hypnosis on your own as it is a powerful mind tool that helps you facilitate change through easy access to the subconscious mind. It easily enables messages to go through the mind and influence your thoughts and actions, in other words your eating and activity habits in a positive way. Its a quick and easy way to teach the mind how to relax so that new suggestions can be introduced thereby reducing, improving and overcoming many negative beliefs and attitudes to create positive changes in your life.

Before you embark on your self-hypnosis journey you:

- o Think about the goals you want to achieve and why you want to achieve them.
- o And keep those goals as realistic as possible, in other words you have to make sure that they are achievable.
- o Think about the time frame you want to achieve your goals.
- o What resources you will need to achieve your goals.
- o What you need to do every day to be able to stay on the right course towards achieving your goals.
- o What problems you need to tackle to achieve your goals
- o What measures you will put into place to make sure that you maintain your goals once you have achieved them.

Breathing in Self-Hypnosis

Deep-breathing in self-hypnosis is very important as it helps you to go into a trance, enables you to stay alert and also deeply relaxes you. Moreover, breathing is a necessity for life.

Correct breathing is crucial in self-hypnosis as it is in everyday health and can be very powerful and effective in the body and mind. Many studies have shown that deeper breathing can relax your body and mind and get rid of stress, help the immune system function better and also signal your body to increase it's metabolism and burn more fat faster. Deep breathing also helps to improve digestion and aids the body in removing excess waste products from the digestive system. Therefore, by improving digestion and eliminating waste products, you begin to lose weight. More so, when your body is stressed your brain tells your adrenal glands to secrete Cortisol, the hormone that signals the fight or flight response also releasing excess insulin which makes the body want to store extra fat and make you crave more sweet and fatty foods, by deep breathing you relax your body and get rid of stress thereby eliminating cortisol, insulin that stimulates excess fat retention. Not only is proper breathing a necessity for self-hypnosis, it has many healthy benefits as well as helping in weight loss!

There are many different breathing exercises or techniques, this is one of them;

o   Find a quiet and comfortable place
o   Any position that is comfortable for you will do as long as you make sure your back is straight
o   Start breathing in relaxing your stomach at the same time as though it's filling with air
o   After filling your stomach with air, keep breathing in and feel your rib cage expand
o   Hold your breath for a moment then begin to breath out slowly
o   As you breath out slowly, relax your chest and rib cage while you pull your stomach in to let the remaining air out
o   Close your eyes and concentrate on your breathing
o   Relax all your body and mind
o   Feel completely relaxed

How to use self-hypnosis
o   Read your script several times before you record it so that you can be very comfortable and used to it.

o Find a place that is quiet and record your script in your normal voice at a relaxed pace, slowing down and softening your voice which will help you to enter hypnosis. You can ask someone to record it for you if you're not comfortable with your voice as there so many people who don't like to hear their own voices. Go with whatever feel natural and right for you.

o Make sure the tone of voice is calm, confident, relaxed, caring, soothing. As you leave hypnosis let the voice return to normal. Beware of background noises such as television, radio, and other noises that will interfere with the hypnosis.

o Do not forget to add a special place into the script if you want it in , this has to be a unique place for you where you can be alone, a place filled with peace and positivity, it can be a place you have visited or an imaginary one, a childhood cherished home with or any other place that relaxes you and is filled with happy memories.

o After recording your script choose a place where you can be completely comfortable and relaxed with no interference, switch your phone, radio, television off. If you choose to sit on a chair make sure that your legs are uncrossed, if you choose to lie down on a couch or bed be aware of not falling asleep halfway through the self-hypnosis process!

o Breath in deeply and out and let your body relax, you can leave your eyes open or close them, breath in and out with each breath feeling your body relax more and more .

o Start your recorded self-hypnosis script and after your session give yourself time to relax and enjoy the calming effect of hypnosis.

o Practice everyday.

Why self-hypnosis?

o Self-hypnosis is empowering and it helps you develop a self-help plan that keeps you in charge and in control of your life. It is very rewarding to know that you can address problems on your own and not rely on other people.

o It promotes self worth and boosts confidence. With self-hypnosis you can re-design and change your script to whatever suits you at any given time based on your choice, needs and what works for you.

o You save a great deal of money with self-hypnosis as well as time, hypnotherapy sessions with a therapist can be very costly.

o Self-hypnosis is also private which can save you embarrassment of sharing private issues that you don't feel comfortable sharing with others. For instance in cases of people who suffer from emotional eating and have past traumatic experiences underlining their emotional eating habits which they don't want to share with anyone, self-hypnosis is a perfect option for them.

Positive thinking

As well as eating healthy and exercising, a positive mental attitude plays a big role in eating healthily and losing weight and makes the process much easier. remember, action starts in the mind!

Positive thinking is basically the act of thinking positively mentally and emotionally. Studies and research show that positive thinking can immensely impact your life and it is often said that we are what we think and that thoughts manifest into things! These statements are reflected accurately in weight loss as positive thinking is a significant tool in weight loss.

Positive thoughts will increase your motivation and energy levels whereas negative thoughts will deflate your motivation and lead to self-defeating behaviours, for example over-eating and stopping exercises.

Focusing on positive aspects of your healthy eating and weight loss plan and how you feel after you have achieved your goal is essential. Think yourself healthy and fit, your ideal weight and believe in yourself and the ability that you will succeed no matter what set-backs come your way. Don't let anything or anyone put you off or bring you down, the trick is not to give up on your ambitions. Your positive mental attitude will carry you a long way through any dilemmas you will encounter. Remember that the way you think tremendously affects the way you feel and act. Your positivity will inspire you to reach your dreams.

Positive statements have to be repeated to your subconscious mind in order for it to programme new ways of thinking, feeling, behaviour and attitudes, they are another way of positive thinking and can be amended anytime that you wish.

Visualization

Visualization is another mind-power mental imagery technique that uses imagination to attain success and bring your desired goal to life. It is like a mental rehearsal aiming to help you to design the life you want for yourself by using imagination and power thoughts, in other words visualization puts you in control.

When you're visualizing be specific and detailed and focus on the positive. Research has found that when your mind enters a state of deep relaxation while visualizing or using other mind techniques, it's very susceptible to any suggestion you give it.

It is paramount that when you're visualizing you shouldn't limit yourself by your beliefs and doubts, the bigger you think and visualize, the greater the opportunity and doors that open to you. Visualization is a very powerful tool for weight loss, healthy eating and exercising, it uses the power of the mind to connect with the body. It is a method used by you, me, celebrities politicians and athletes to attain our personal goals and if you think that it's all a rubbish then you're very wrong because a lot of research has proven visualization to be very effective if its practiced regularly. Visualization focuses your mind and thoughts and feelings towards your perfect weight hence by visualizing and imagining yourself as being healthy with your desired weight you will make your subconscious mind believe that you're slim and healthy and therefore you will start to behave and act according to this new image that it holds in your mind. To achieve your weight loss goals through visualization, you need to:

o Set your intentions for losing weight
o Hold a mental picture of your desired outcome in your mind
o Imagine how you will feel after you have achieved your goals
o Visualize yourself acting in a way reflecting your healthy and perfect weight

- Be positive throughout all your visualization and avoid any negative thinking, don't give in to any conflicts and doubts in your mind. Your chances of achieving your goals will be greater with positive thinking.

Meditation

Meditation is the act of focussing, silencing and clearing the mind of any thoughts and doesn't have to be complicated. It is very simple and easy but requires time, discipline and dedication. It is about being in the present and it facilitates healthy and productive thinking.

When you discipline your mind you will be calm, relaxed and aware of your feelings, thoughts and emotions. An undisciplined mind reacts easily to anger, frustration, fear, nerves and confusion. Meditation is a technique that gives you a key to self-awareness that can be useful in many areas of your life. It teaches you to be in control of your mind and emotions. In meditation the mind slows down and you are able to see the things you worry about, fear or are angry about, frustrations, obsessions, doubts, conflicts and confusion within us and it's in meditation that we learn to break this pattern by working through the thoughts that come up and then rejecting them. When you meditate all negativity comes up and the emotions attached to those negative feelings. For people who have a problem with emotional eating, meditation gets you in touch with what's going on inside your mind and you begin to recognize what exactly is causing your problems and the emotions underlying your cravings for food. A lot of time people over-eat because of stress, by meditating you release stress and will no longer comfort eat. Meditation will help you relax and thereby increasing your self-awareness, so you're less likely to indulge in emotional eating.

Meditation technique is helpful in a way that it supports your healthy eating plan and also your weight loss by getting in touch with your feelings, emotions and thoughts towards food. Meditation is not a religion but rather a way of listening to the universe, your higher self, God or whatever you call it. Meditations is not hypnosis either, hypnosis is about the mind and thought, whereas meditation goes further than that. People assume that meditation is a very hard task without even trying in many cases, because it is to do with silencing the mind. Because as humans we are driven by our thoughts, emotions and egos hence questioning and analysing everything that goes through our minds making it hard for the mind to stop and recharge. Most people who are starting out to meditate will find it extremely hard to silence the mind, often referred to as the "monkey mind" or "chatter mind" as thoughts will keep popping in and out of the mind constantly. For meditation to take full effect you have to persevere no matter how busy your mind gets, when a thought comes forward accept it and allow yourself to feel whatever emotions are coming up, then let the thought go and so forth and with time your mind will learn to slow down and bring less of these thoughts up as you work through them daily. And as you continue to practice your meditation everyday your mind will eventually learn to be still for lengthy periods which will allow you to reach deeper levels of unconsciousness where you will be able to work through whatever issues you want to work on and change on a deeper emotional level. By meditating you can liberate yourself from everything that is holding you back, for instance fears, negative emotions and feelings, anxieties, pain from past traumas, and negative beliefs.

If you find it hard to meditate on your own for various reasons then you should try and join a meditation group. Meditating in a group will motivate you to keep going and you will also get support from others.

Breathing as a part of meditation is very important as you focus your attention on it, it will help to distract you from your thoughts and getting caught up in your delusions and conflicts. Breathing will help you to settle into a deeper relaxation and stillness as it is not attached to any emotion and you can easily control it as you want.

There is no right or wrong way to meditate;

- o Start off small with one minute, three minutes, five minutes and so forth until your mind has got the hang of it. It may take time but you will get there
- o Meditate your own way, do whatever feels comfortable for you
- o Find a quiet and peaceful place
- o You can either lie down or sit down
- o Meditation takes practice and patience
- o However hard it may be to quiet and still your mind at first, as thoughts will keep popping in and out, you

have to be persistent don't give up and soon your mind will be trained to stay still and then you will reap the benefits.

o   Hold a mental picture of you looking healthy at your ideal weight
o . Be positive

Relaxation Technique

Relaxation is essential to body and mind as it is linked to a higher level of feel good chemicals such as Serotin. Scientific studies have proved that deep relaxation can have a big impact on a wide range of medical conditions. Relaxation brings about a state of calmness, rest, the muscles relax, food is digested, the heart beat slows down, blood circulation flows freely through the body and it also brings about renewal mentally and physically.

Relaxation is an important part of your weight loss plan. Given that stress is often one of the factors that make people over-eat and gain weight, being able to relax is one of the most powerful tools to losing weight and staying fit and healthy. Experts believe that reducing stress stops craving for fatty and sweet foods by learning and practicing relaxation techniques as part of the weight loss plan greatly increases the effectiveness of managing stress and emotions without feeling the need to resort to unhealthy eating.

Relaxation exercise can be used prior to meditation and visualisation for the purpose of going into a deep relaxation in order to connect with the subconscious mind.

Stress affects your body in many ways for instance;

- o Behavioural- You eat more when you're stressed using food as a comforter or clutch.
- o Hormonal- Chronic stress raises the blood level of Cortisol, then cortisol raises your blood sugar and causes fat cells to grow larger. High levels of Cortisol increases your amount of belly fat and it also increases food consumption particularly fatty and sweet foods by turning off your brain's natural appetite - suppressing signals, therefore a good reason to relax as relaxation will aid with your weight loss.

The following are the scientifically proven benefits of relaxation;

- o It boosts immunity
- o It boosts fertility
- o Lowers blood pressure
- o Slows heart rate
- o Reduces muscle tension
- o Reduces inflammation in arthritis, asthma and skin conditions like psoriasis
- o It reduces stress and anxiety
- o Lifts depressed moods

Relaxation technique

Close your eyes and sit back comfortably with your feet together .... hands resting on the sides of the chair or on your thighs .... take a nice deep breath and begin to relax ..... breath in again and hold your breath ...... then let go of it and feel yourself letting go of all the stress and tension as you breath out ...... just think about relaxing every muscle in your body from your head to your toes ...... and keep breathing deeply in and out ...... feeling the calm and relaxation flowing through your body relaxing you all over .... every time you breath in and out you become more and more relaxed ...... now think about nothing else but how your body feels ..... continuing to breath in and out ...... now focus on the muscles around your eyes and around your mouth ...... let them relax ...... and the muscles in your jaw are completely relaxed too .....feel them relax even more as you drift and float into a deeper level of relaxation ...... let the muscles in your neck and shoulders relax ...... feeling you with soothing relaxation .... the relaxation spreads to muscles in your back ...... running down your arms and your finger tips as you continue to breath in and out feeling completely relaxed .... now I want you to notice this same feeling moving to your chest, stomach and thighs ...... you breath in and relax these muscles and as you breath out you relax the muscles in your legs .... to the tips of your toes .... your whole body is covered with a complete sense of relaxation ..... you are floating deeper .... and deeper ....Now count from one to five and as you count from one to five ...... you will let yourself sink more and more deeply into this nice relaxed state ...... One ..... deeper and deeper ...... Two ...... you feel more and more relaxed ..... Three ..... you are sinking deeper and deeper ...... Four ...... you feel so heavy and relaxed ..... Five ...... Now that you're so deeply relaxed ...... imagine yourself in your special place ...... a place that means a lot to you and makes you feel loved, happy, calm and at peace

...... feel it and imagine it ...... enjoy these tranquil feelings and keep them with you ...... allow these feelings to grow stronger and stronger and spread through your body and mind ..... you feel good inside and out in this place ...... with a sense of tremendous well-being surrounding you ...... and these positive feelings will remain with you for a long time ......

You can remain in this relaxed state as long as you wish ...... when you're ready count from one to five ...... slowly feeling your body returning to its normal state ...... and your mind becoming more alert ...... on the count of five you will open your eyes and you will feel relaxed, calm and wonderful ......

****

Part Two

HEALTHY EATING AND THE MIND

The power that the mind has over our well-being is incredible and immense. When you consistently think about something, you're bringing it to life and creating it because thought is real and powerful. Therefore the ability to train your mind to think healthy will help you a great deal in achieving your goals. Not only is the power of your mind responsible for your eating habits and choices, it also plays a big role in your weight loss and maintenance. You just have to learn to train your mind to change the way you think, feel and act around food. For instance change your bad eating habits into healthy ones by changing your thought pattern. That is to say when you think about healthy food and how it will nourish, energize and keep you fit as well as losing weight, you will find yourself making a choice of healthy foods and eating healthily. Hence its vital that you work with your subconscious mind when making food choices as a trained mind will always make a choice of nutritious healthy foods.

NUTRITION

Nutrition is the process of providing the food necessary for health and growth. The essential nutrients for life include carbohydrates, proteins, fats, vitamins and minerals. The human body is 63% water, 22% proteins, 13% fat and 2% minerals. A healthy balanced diet is one that gives your body the nutrients it needs to function properly. Basically you are what you eat, whatever goes into your body either strengthens and nourishes it or weakens it, therefore its crucial to eat the right foods- a balanced diet can determine how you look, feel and act. The key to a healthy balanced diet is eating the right amount of food for how active we are and eating a variety of nutritious food. It is therefore important to remember that you eat to live and not live to eat and that food should be part of life that should not to be abused or obsessed about. In other words we should aim at having a healthy relationship with food.

Proteins

Proteins are large molecules consisting of amino acids which our bodies and cells in our bodies need to function properly. Our body's structures, functions and regulation of tissues, cells and organs cannot exist without proteins. Protein is found throughout the body in muscles, skin, bones, hair. Many other parts also contain significant amounts of protein.

Enzymes, hormones and antibodies are proteins. Protein accounts for 20% of total body weight. A proper balanced diet provides enough protein without the need for protein supplements.

Sources of proteins; Eggs, fish and sea food, milk, cheese, yogurt, white meat, chicken, turkey, lean pork, lean beef, beans, peas, soy products, nuts and seeds, sorghum, millet.

Functions of proteins
o   Enzymes are proteins that facilitate biochemical reactions.

32

o Anti-bodies and enzymes are proteins produced by the immune system to help remove foreign substances and fight infections

o DNA - associated proteins regulate chromosome structure during cell division and play a role in regulating gene expression.

o Structural protein provide support in our bodies, for example proteins in our connective tissues such as collagen and elastin.

o Contractile proteins are involved in muscle contraction and movement for example actin and myocin.

o Hormone proteins co-ordinate bodily functions, for instance insulin controls our blood-sugar concentration by regulating the uptake of glucose into cells. Also proteins transport molecules around the body for example haemoglobin transports oxygen through the blood.

Lack of protein in the body can cause;

o Muscle wastage or shrinkage
o Oedema- Fluid building up in feet and ankles
o Anaemia
o Slow growth in children
o Hair loss
o Reduced energy levels
o Frequent infections
o Mental problems
o Skin problems
o Weight loss
o Low blood pressure

Carbohydrates

Carbohydrates are sugars that break down inside the body to create glucose. Glucose is moved around the body in the blood and is the primary source of energy for the brain.

Carbohydrates are the most important source of energy for the body and are found in almost all living things and play a vital role in the proper functioning of the immune system, fertilization, blood clotting and human development. There are two types of carbohydrates, simple and complex depending on their chemical structure. Simple carbohydrates include sugars found naturally in fruit, vegetables, milk and milk products and also include sugars added during food processing and refining where as complex carbohydrates on the other hand include wholegrain breads, cereals, starchy vegetables and legumes. Excess consumption of carbohydrates can lead to weight gain, types 2 diabetes and cancer.

Sources of carbohydrates

- Grain products- wheat, oats, rice, cornmeal, millet, sorghum, brown pasta, cereals, whole-wheat bread
- Starchy vegetables and beans- potatoes, cassava, yam, green bananas, corn, green peas, dry beans
- Leafy green vegetables- Spinach, cabbage, broccoli
- Fruit and fruit juices contain carbohydrates in the form of natural sugars such as glucose and fructose.
- Beverages- Diary milk, sugar sweetened soda, fruit drinks, sports energy drinks, wine, beer and liqueurs
- Sweets and added sugar

Functions of carbohydrates

o Energy supply, particularly for the brain in the form of glucose
o Protein sparing action- used for energy and sparing proteins for tissue building and repairing
o Essential for fat oxidation
o Plays an important role in the gas to – intestinal function
o Adds flavour to the diet- easily digested and forms the staple food for human beings
o Cellular and protein recognition
o Dietary fibre for the body

Carbohydrate deficiency in the body may cause;

o Fatigue and weakness- decreased energy levels
o Hypoglycemia- lack of glucose
o Muscle wasting
o Unhealthy weight loss- losing fat and muscle
o Dehydration and reduced body secretions
o Loss of sodium- leading to clumps and exhaustion
o Weakened immune system
o Constipation- due to inadequate fibre in the body
o Mood swings and depression as brains stops regulating serotin hormone
o Acidosis- increased acid in the body due to low-carbohydrate diet
o Ketosis- which is caused by lack of enough glucose for energy in the body

Fats

Fat is a nutrient that is essential for normal body function. Fats play diverse roles in human nutrition. They are important as a source of energy both for immediate utilization by the body and in laying down a storage depot for later utilization when food intake is reduced.

Fat is an essential part of our diet and nutrition, therefore we all need fat in our daily food intake, but too much of a particular kind of fat called saturated fat can raise our cholesterol, which increases the risk of heart disease. Its important to cut down on fat and chose foods that contain unsaturated fats.

There are two types of fat which are saturated fats and unsaturated fats, unsaturated fats can be mono-saturated or poly-saturated.

- o Mono-saturated fats are healthy fats- examples are olive oil, peanut oil, avocado oil, nuts and seeds and un hydrogenated margarines
- o Poly-saturated fats are also healthy fats- examples are omega 6 fat- sesame oil, sunflower oil, corn oils, non-hydrogenated margarines, nuts and seeds. Omega 3 fats- Fattier fish, canola oils, soy bean oils, flax seed, omega 3 eggs, walnuts
- o Saturated fats are un-healthy fats- found in foods prepared with hydrogenated oils as well as fatty meats, full fat diary products, butter, lard, coconut oil, palm oil, palm kernel, cocoa butter, snack foods, fast food, in all foods made with shortening or particularly hydrogenated vegetable oils and ready prepared foods.

Functions of fats

o To provide energy- Although the main source of energy in our bodies is carbohydrates, fat is used as a source of backup energy in cases when carbohydrates are not available.
o To absorb certain nutrients
o Maintain body temperature- to keep warm
o Good fats protect the heart and keep the body healthy

Lack of fats in the body can lead to;

o Achy joints
o Cold intolerance symptoms
o Cracked dry skin
o Eczema
o Excessive thirst
o Gastro-intestinal problems
o Hypertension
o Constipation due to Irregular bowel movements
o Weakness
o Low concentration
o Low mental energy
o Low body weight
o Poor memory
o Poor wound healing
o Symptoms of hyperactivity

Vitamins and minerals

Vitamins and minerals are essential nutrients that our bodies need in small amounts to function properly. There are two types of vitamins : Fat-soluble vitamins and Water-soluble vitamins.

Fat-soluble vitamins are vitamins A, D, E and K, they are found mainly in fatty foods and animal products, these vitamins dissolve in fat and are stored in the body tissues.

Water-soluble vitamins are vitamins C, B, and Folic acid, they are found in a many different kinds of foods including fruit and vegetables. Unlike the fat-soluble vitamins, water-soluble vitamins dissolve in water and therefore can be easily lost in water while cooking and heat can also damage them too. So the best way to prepare them and preserving their nutrient content is by steaming or grilling.

MINERALS

The body needs several minerals and a balanced diet should provide all the essential minerals. They are divided into two groups which are major minerals (macro minerals) and trace minerals (micro minerals). Major minerals are; Sodium, chloride, potassium, calcium, phosphorus, magnesium, sulphur. Macro minerals are; Iron, zinc, iodine, fluoride, manganese. Other micro minerals are copper, selenium, chromium and molybdenum.

Importance of vitamins and minerals in the body

- o For strong bones- calcium, vitamin D, vitamin K, magnesium and phosphorus protect bones against fractures
- o Healthy teeth- fluoride helps bone formation and keeps cavities from decaying

o Preventing birth defects- taking folic acid early in the early stages of pregnancy prevents brain and spinal birth defects in babies
o Help with energy production in the body- vitamin B1, and B2
o Help maintain a healthy immune system- vitamin E and magnesium
o Important for vision- vitamin A
o Play a big role in blood clotting- vitamin K
o For proper fluid balance, nerve transmission and muscle contraction- sodium, chloride and potassium.

Lack of vitamins and minerals may cause;

o Scurvy- lack of vitamin C
o Rickets and osteoporosis- caused by lack of vitamin D, calcium
o Beriberi- lack of vitamin B1
o Pellagra- vitamin B3 deficiency
o Anaemia- Lack of iron, folic acid
o Weak bones and teeth- lack of fluoride

Dietary fibre or Roughage

Fibre is an essential nutrient required for a proper digestive track and it fills you up too. A lack of fibre in your diet can lead to constipation, haemorrhoids and raised levels of cholesterol and blood sugar. However excess fibre can lead to bowel obstruction, diarrhoea and even dehydration. If you increase your fibre intake, you should also drink more water.

Eating more fibre in your diet will not only keep you lean and healthy but also help you lose weight and maintain it. Hence high fibre foods take longer to eat and they fill you up leaving you full and satisfied and they also lower levels of insulin, the appetite stimulating hormone. Also when you eat high fibre foods more calories are used during digestion and absorption of high-fibre foods, and lastly high fibre foods are lower in calories and therefore help you keep healthy, lose weight and control the weight loss.

Examples of high fibre foods;

- o Fresh fruit- Apples, pears, guava, kiwi
- o Mangoes, oranges, blueberries, blackberries
- o Dates, figs, avocado, banana, raspberries
- o Prunes
- o Dried fruit- Figs, raisins, apricots, dates extra
- o Potatoes, sweet potatoes, yams with skin
- o Fruit juices with pulp
- o Lentils- beans, green peas, chickpeas
- o Whole grains and cereals
- o Vegetables- Carrots, broccoli, Brussels
- o sprouts, cabbage, spinach, rhubarb extra
- o Nuts- Almonds, walnuts, pecans
- o Seeds

Water

Water is an essential part of our everyday diet, vital for our well being. Your body needs plenty of water to be able to function properly and the body cannot function without it as every cell in the body needs water.

The body is made up of 50-75% of water with the brain consisting of 90% water, muscle 75%, bone 22%, blood 83%. The body can't store water so we need fresh supplies of it everyday to make up for losses from urine, urine and faeces.

Benefits of drinking water

o Lose weight-water flushes down by-products of fat, reduces hunger, is an effective appetite suppressant. In other words when you drink more water you eat less and plus water has no calories

o Water is a natural remedy for headaches given the fact that dehydration is one of the causes of headaches

o It improves exercise as your body's temperature is regulated efficiently so you will feel more energetic with water fuelling your muscles

o Your brain works more efficiently with plenty of water, concentration and alertness is immensely boosted

o Drinking water helps in digestion and prevents constipation, for efficient bowel movement you need plenty of water and fibre

o Water in your body helps keep your joints and muscles lubricated hence preventing sprains and cramps during exercise and playing sports

o Water relives fatigue and lifts your moods

o Water moisturises and increases skin elasticity leading to a healthy skin.

Importance of water in the body

o It transports nutrients and oxygen into cells
o Maintains health and integrity of every cell in the body
o Helps eliminate by-products of the body such as urine, sweet and faeces
o Regulates body's temperature through sweating
o Water aids digestion and prevents constipation
o Helps with metabolism
o Detoxifies our bodies
o Serves as a shock absorber inside the eyes, spinal cord and in the amniotic sac surrounding the foetus in pregnancy
o Lubricates and cushions the joints
o Moisturises the skin to maintain its texture and appearance.

Effects and symptoms of dehydration

o Tiredness
o Migraine
o Constipation
o Muscle cramps
o Irregular blood pressure
o Dry skin
o Kidney problems
o Risk of death if a person is 20% dehydrated

What is a calorie?

A calorie in scientific terms is a unit of heat and the energy producing property for food. The idea is that if the number of calories going into your body are less than the calories being used up by bodily activity and exercise, then you will lose weight.

Calories in food

Knowing your calorie intake in food can be useful in aiding you to staying healthy and maintaining a healthy weight. It helps you to keep track of the amount of energy you're eating and that you're not consuming more than you should. Most packages of food state calorie content on the nutrition label, this information is often given in kcals which is a short term for "kilocalories" and also in KJ which is short for " "kilojoules".

A kilocalorie is another term for calorie so 2000 calories will be written as 2000kcals. Kilojoules are the metric measurement of calories. To find the energy content in kilojoules, multiply the calorie by 4.2.

Crash diets and 'yoyo' dieting

When you diet you drain yourself mentally, physically and emotionally. You should stay clear of all forms of diets because they cause feelings of anger and resentment within you as food becomes an enemy and guilt which can lead to a number of eating disorders for example bulimia and anorexia. It is commonly known that most diets don't work as people tend to go on them, lose weight and then pile it all back on and more, it is very un-healthy to lose weight this way because it destroys your attitude to food and normal eating pattern. The only way to lose weight healthily is by having the right mental attitude or mind power, eating healthy, and keeping active. The human body works like a car if you put diesel in a petrol car it will not work, you will need the right fuel for it to run smoothly!

There are so many diets, probably hundreds, and more keep popping up everyday, but the truth is that they don't work. If they did work in the first place there wouldn't be any need for new ones and the rate of people who are overweight and obese would have gone down!

Moreover after the end of your crash diet you will go back to your normal pattern of eating with a slower metabolism and regaining all the weight that you lost and worse still putting on even more in the process. In addition, diets often contradict themselves which makes it harder and confusing for the people who use them. The truth is that you have to take your power back and decide what is right for you and what is not. It is common sense that a new way of thinking, a new way of eating and keeping active is the only natural and sensible way for permanent results.

Diets don't work because they are temporary and therefore the results are short lived too. Maintaining health and losing weight should be a long-term measure which in return will yield long lasting results. When you're dieting your brain will tell your body that you're starving hence giving the impression that food is scarce and by doing so, slows down the metabolism to utilise the small amount of food available as best as possible.

Dieting is the greatest risk factor for developing an eating disorder as most weight loss diets are very restrictive and leave the people who are dieting excruciatingly hungry, therefore the ensuing starving and binge eating eventually results in eating disorders. Among which are:

Anorexia nervosa- this is an eating disorder where the person starves themselves in order to lose weight or they exercise excessively. Anorexia often starts as dieting and affects both body and mind. People with anorexia become dangerously thin but in their mind they view and see themselves as fat.

Bulimia nervosa- is another eating disorder that is characterized by bouts of constant binge eating followed by forced vomiting, taking laxatives or diuretics in order to get rid of the food and calories and prevent weight gain. Bulimia like anorexia may start as dieting and then progresses into a cycle.

Binge eating disorder- is a serious mental illness where people eat very large amounts of food over a short period of time often in private. Unlike bulimia, people who suffer from binge eating disorder don't make themselves vomit after eating. Binge eating often leads to feelings of guilt, embarrassment, anxiety and low self-esteem because of their lack of controlling their eating habit. Binge eating may also start as a diet, which leads to periods of starvation followed by binge eating.

What is Metabolism?

Your metabolism is the total of all the calorie burning changes that occur in the body. Your resting metabolism rate (RMR) is the amount of calories you burn when you're completely resting. Age, size, gender and genes all play an important part in determining your metabolism. Men have a faster metabolic rate than women because they have more muscle mass, heavier bones and less body fat than women. And with age people gain more fat and lose muscle therefore their body mass rate decreases. Genes also play a role in muscle size, bone density and ability to grow muscle which all affect metabolism.

Further more, exercise, body temperature, hormone changes and digestion all increase the metabolism rate.

Metabolism and digestion

Our metabolic rate increases during food digestion, this is why it is important to eat little and often rather than eating a few large meals with long breaks in between the consumption of a meal. The constant work by your body to go through the digestion process of the breakdown of food keeps your metabolism active, thus increasing the metabolic rate.

Body Mass Index (BMI)

Is the measurement of healthy weight based on your height and weight. BMI gives you an idea of whether you're under weight, a healthy weight, over weight or obese. For example the BMI of a gentleman aged 39 weighing 70kg and measures 1.75m in height is worked out as follows;

BMI= weight in pounds divided by height in inches squared or weight in kilograms divided by height in meters squared.

Divide 70 by 1.75= 40

Then divide 40 by 1.75= 22.9

His BMI = 22.9 which is in the normal range.

Underweight: BMI less than 18.5

Healthy weight: BMI is 18.5 to 24.9

Over weight: BMI is 25 to 29.9

Obese: BMI is 30 or higher

NOTE: Even if your BMI falls in the normal weight category, you will still have a high risk of ill-health if you smoke, don't exercise regularly and eat lots of food lacking in nutrients with high sugar, fat content and salt.

See Table overleaf.

Body Mass Index(BMI)

**Weight
in pounds   Height (feet, inches)**

	5'0	5'3	5'6	5'9	6'0	6'3
140	27	25	23	21	19	18
150	29	27	24	22	20	19
160	31	28	26	24	22	20
170	33	30	28	25	23	21
180	35	32	29	27	25	23
190	37	34	31	28	26	24
200	39	36	32	30	27	25
210	41	37	34	31	29	26
220	42	39	36	33	30	28
230	45	41	37	34	21	39
240	47	43	39	36	33	30
250	49	44	40	37	34	31

Fat, sugar and salt

Although fat, sugar and salt are essential for your body to function properly, they should be eaten in small amounts as too much consumption is detrimental to health. Fat, sugar and salt are contained in high amounts in processed foods, savoury snacks and ready meals.

Eating a balanced diet that is high in fruit, vegetables, fibre, water and low in fat, sugar and salt will help you to maintain good health and also lose weight. It is also very important that you cook your own meals as often as you can as this is the best way to make sure that you're eating the best and highest quality nutrients that your body needs.

Fat and health

Your body makes its own fat from the excess calories that you eat, this fat is important to your health for a number of your body's functions. But you have to be careful when choosing which fat to eat as some fats are un-healthy, and even with the healthy fat you have to keep your consumption moderate. Fat is high in calories, if you eat more calories than you need, you will put on weight. Un-healthy dietary fats are; Saturated fat which is a form of fat that comes from mainly animal sources of food such as red meat, poultry and full fat dairy products. Another un-healthy fat is trans fat which occurs naturally in some foods in small amounts. But most trans fats are made from oils through a food processing method called partial hydrogenation. Healthier dietary fat are;

o   Mono-saturated fat found in a variety of foods and oils. Polyunsaturated fat is found in plant –based foods and oils. Omega-3 o Fatty acids- found in some types of fatty fish like salmon, sardines, trout, mackerel, herring, pilchards, fresh tuna.

A diet high in fat is damaging and could cause;

o Diabetes- is directly linked to high fat diets and obesity. Diabetes leads to high blood pressure which then can cause numerous health ailments including renal failure and cardiovascular disease.

o Fat filled diets can contribute to excessive wear and tear on your joints, putting you at risk of developing arthritis conditions. It can also cause bone fractures.

o Stroke- Diets that are high in fat increase blood pressure. Fat constricts your arteries making it very difficult for blood to flow throughout the body and brain hence causing stroke.

o Heart conditions-foods high in fat are high in cholesterol, this excess fat blocks your coronary arteries leading to a heart attack.

o Cancer- Eating a diet high in fat will increase your chances of developing cancer.

o Alcoholic Liver Disease- caused by too much fat in the liver as a result of drinking large amounts of alcohol (high in calories- fat).

Tips on cutting down on fat

o Read the product nutrition label and go for the non- fat, low fat or reduced fat content products o Stick to lean meats with no skin or fat on

o Avoid saturate oils when cooking such as butter and lard, opt for oils high in mono-un-saturates like olive oil and sunflower oil which is high in poly-unsaturates

o Use low fat milk, yogurts and spreads

o Use low fat cheese or mayonnaise on sandwiches rather than butter or spreads

o Try and cook your food from scratch which will make it easier for you to control the amount of fat that goes in.

o Grill your meats rather than frying them

o Cut down on high fat foods when eating out or ordering takeaways, go for the low fat healthier options for instance grilled, steamed, salad meals

o Cut down on your alcohol intake.

Sugar and health

Added sugar is harmful to the body and health and also contributes to many illnesses. Sugar is an empty substance and contains no nutrients, proteins, enzymes or healthy fats on its own. The best form of sugar for your health is the natural sugar found in fruit and vegetables which is packed with fibre, vitamins and enzymes.

Added sugar is harmful to health in the following ways:

o It increases bad cholesterol

o Contributes to weight gain

o Causes sugar addiction in the brain

o Added sugar encourages you to eat more as it doesn't fill you up

o It causes tooth decay. Decay happens when sugar reacts with the bacteria in plaque. This forms the acids that attack the teeth and destroy the enamel, when this happens repeatedly the tooth enamel starts to break down forming a hole or cavity into the tooth leading to the tooth decaying quickly

o Eating too much sugar will impair your immune system and affect your body's ability to fight off illnesses. Also drinking high sugar sweetened beverages can raise blood pressure

o Diabetes- the more sugar you eat, the more fluctuations you will have in your blood sugar levels.

o Consuming too much sugar will increase your insulin levels and put you at risk of chronic diseases for example heart disease, some cancers, polycystic ovarian syndrome among others.

o A binge on sugar can also impact your mental health in form of depression.

Tips on cutting down on sugar

o Read the nutrition labels on the packaging and know what sugar content is in the food you're buying. Look out for other terms used for sugar on labels like Maltose, molasses, honey, invert sugar corn syrup or hydrolysed starch. There is always a colour coded nutrition information indicating whether sugar is low, medium or high. Green is for low, amber for medium and red for high sugar content.

o Swap sugary drinks for water, if you're craving something sweet eat fruit as fruit is a healthy option packed with natural sugars.

o Buy un-sweetened food products.

o Go for plain porridge or cereal products.

o Avoid drinking soft drinks as they are high in sugar, drink water instead or go for the sugar free drinks.

o Reduce sugar in your tea or coffee or cut it out completely and go sugar free.

o Avoid cereals coated in sugar.

o When ordering takeaways or eating out be aware of foods that are high in sugar for instance sweet chilli, curry sauces, and some salad dressings that are high in sugar.

o Eat healthier snacks that don't contain high sugar quantities for example fruit, unsalted nuts, oat cakes extra.

Salt and health

Although salt benefits your health immensely in various ways, too much consumption can be problematic. According to the National Health Service (NHS) adults should not be eating more that 6g of salt and that salt levels should be even much lower that this for babies and children. These are a few examples of the foods that are high in salt: bacon, ham, anchovies, pickles, prawns, salami, salted nuts, salt fish, smoked meat and fish, soy sauce, stock cubes, and yeast extract. Research shows that a high intake of salt can lead to;

o High blood pressure
o Stroke-high blood pressure is the single major factor responsible for stroke and salt is the major factor responsible for many of these strokes.
o Coronary Heart Disease- is a condition when the heart's blood supply is reduced or blocked leading to heart failure and heart attacks. Raised high blood pressure is the major risk factor for CHD and high blood pressure is caused by high salt intake.
o High salt intake causes weight gain- obesity.
o Water retention- high salt intake causes the body to retain water.
o Studies have shown that a diet high in salt can worsen asthma.
o High levels of salt in the body can raise the risk of developing diabetes by raising blood pressure.
o Kidney stones and kidney disease- are also a common problem with people who consume vast amounts of salt. A high salt intake and high blood pressure can cause too much calcium to be excreted by the kidneys into the urine, leading to a build up of calcium which forms into kidney stones which are extremely painful. Furthermore a high salt intake can disrupt the function of the kidneys and cause high blood pressure and by doing so putting a strain on the kidneys causing kidney disease.

o Because most calcium in the body is stored in the bones, a diet high in salt causes calcium to be lost from the bones and excreted in the urine, making the bones weak and easily broken hence osteoporosis.

o Stomach cancer- a high salt diet increases the risk of stomach cancer which makes it more vulnerable to bacteria (H.Pylori)

Tips on cutting down on salt

o Check the food nutrition labels and look out for sodium chloride which is another term used for salt on the labels.

o You need to be aware of the salt that is already in the foods you buy. As with sugar there is always a colour coded nutrition information indicating whether salt is low, medium or high. Green for low (0.3g or less per 100g), amber for medium and red for high (1.5g salt per 100g)

o Buy reduced salt foods.

o Avoid high processed foods.

o Don't add salt to food when cooking.

o Replace crisps with healthier snacks like fruit, vegetable sticks or un-salted nuts.

o Try to cook with vegetables as they contain natural salt.

o Cut back on processed meats and consume fresh ones which naturally contain salt.

o Compare various brands and go for the ones with lowest salt content.

o Add spices to your cooking, they contain natural salt and also add flavour to your food.

Causes of weight gain

o Over-eating – when you consume more calories than you can burn consistently, you will gain weight. Inevitably binge eating and continuing to eat when you're full or not hungry will do the damage.

o Lack of exercise- if you take those calories without getting active to burn them off then you are very like to gain weight and at risk of many health risks linked to lack of exercise like obesity, coronary heart disease, high blood pressure among others.

o Food addiction- this is addiction to junk food, foods high in sugar, fats and salt trigger feel good brain chemicals such as dopamine, hence as soon as you finish eating and the pleasure that you've experienced while eating wanes off, you will have the urge to continue eating so that you can experience the pleasure again, so the eating pattern carries on and on despite lots of weight gain.

o Chronic stress- when you're stressed, your body produces chemical substances like cortisol hormone that makes your body more likely to store fat especially around the waist. This type of weight increases your risk of serious health problems.

o Hypothyroidism- happens when the thyroid is under active, the body doesn't produces enough thyroid hormone to help burn stored fat. This causes the metabolism to slow down and store more fat than you can burn especially when you're not physically active.

o Genetics- According to research, there is a link to genetics and weight gain and that "fat" genes can be inherited from parents as well as inheriting their bad un-healthy habits such as un-healthy eating, over-eating and lack of activity.

o Polycystic Ovary Syndrome (PCOS)- is a disease caused by a result of hormonal imbalance, it causes weight gain without excessive eating.

o Depression- a vast number of people turn to eating when they are depressed in order to ease their mental and emotional pain.

o Cushing's Syndrome- caused when the adrenal glands produce too much cortisol, which leads to a build up of fat in the face, upper back and abdomen.

o Syndrome X- also called insulin resistance, it is linked to weight gain, when your body is resistant to the hormone insulin, other hormones that control your metabolism don't work as well. Hence weight gain.

o Hormonal changes in women- because women have frequent changes of hormones in their bodies, for instance puberty, menstruation cycle, pregnancy and menopause, this may cause over-eating and weight gain.

o Medication- Certain medicines are often linked to weight gain, these include; diabetes medicines, steroids and hormones (HRT) for arthritis and similar conditions, some over the counter medicines, depression and mental illness drugs, anti-convulsants for epilepsy and other neurological conditions, some heart and blood pressure medicines, contraceptive pills, beta blockers for migraines and high blood pressure, allergy medications such as antihistamines and corticosteroids.

o Insomnia
o Food allergies

Why people over-eat

The following are the most common reasons why people over-eat.

o Stress- eating because they are stressed and food helps them to relax but only temporarily.
o To reward themselves- for attaining a big goal or a just a simple task.
o For entertainment- because they're bored so eating in front of the television or at the cinema becomes a habit.
o Wanting to be noticed- seeking attention and wanting to be and maybe even look different by over-eating and gaining excessive amounts of weight.
o Eating to cut out negative past experiences for example an
o abusive childhood, thereby using food as a comforter.
o Eating because of fear or insecurities for example a woman may overeat to gain weight and ward off any attention from men, this is mostly common in women who were abused as children therefore they hold a

negative view of men. Also a husband or boyfriend may encourage his wife or girlfriend to overeat because he's insecure and scared that if she looks slim and attractive, she will leave him for other men.

o Some people seek love in food such as by over-eating they are giving themselves the love that they can't get elsewhere.

Emotional eating

Emotional eating is consuming a vast amount of food to relieve negative feelings and emotions rather than suppressing hunger. Research and studies estimate that 75% of over-eating is caused by emotions. A lot of people perceive that food brings or at least can bring them comfort, so they end up over-eating mostly comfort junk foods with low nutrition value for example chips, cookies, cake, chocolate extra. Eating becomes a habit to fill the emotional void and also mask the problems behind and actually prevents them from being able to take action and address their emotional distress.

What causes emotional eating?

o Depression
o Stress
o Boredom
o Loneliness
o Abusive relationships
o Childhood traumas

o Low self-esteem
o Anger
o Anxiety
o Bullying
o Financial problems
o Illness
o Sadness

Emotional eating triggers can be;

o Social- eating around other people or being encouraged by other people to eat or eating to fit into a group.
o Emotional stress- eating to fill the void or escape whatever problems are causing the stress.
o Situational- eating because there is an opportunity to do so for example Christmas, wedding, party, cinema, family gatherings, restaurant or when watching television.
o Negative thoughts and feelings of low self-worth and esteem can also trigger emotional eating.
o Physiological- eating in response to the body's demands for instance if a person has been dieting or missing meals, they will go on a food binge after the dieting phase.

Overcoming emotional eating

The first step to managing emotional eating is the sufferer learning healthier ways to view food, establish healthy eating and identifying what triggers their emotional eating and also learn ways to alleviate stress with self-hypnosis, relaxation techniques, deep breathing techniques, meditation and exercising. These can all have tremendous benefits to health and alleviating stress.

- o It is important that you avoid any activities or substances that will worsen the problem or prevent you from dealing with it for instance using drugs or alcohol.
- o Develop alternatives to un-healthy eating habits for example rather than sitting around eating and mulling over negative thoughts; go for a walk or jog, meditate, use the relaxation technique, listen to music, read a book, call a friend, do some gardening or housework, join a group or club and meet with the same interests as you, do some charity work! Helping other people will raise your spirits and boost your self-worth.
- o Stay away from people who encourage your eating and keep the company of people who inspire you.
- o Try and keep a positive mind, plenty of exercise will lift your moods
- o An eating pattern exercise will help you to examine in detail your eating pattern and also to identify when you're most likely to eat, where you eat and why you eat.

Despite the causes of your eating, you will have to replace the emotional satisfaction that food gives you with an activity that provides you with the same feeling.

Eating Pattern Exercise See overleaf.

When

I eat when I am	Bored	Yes	No
	Stressed	Yes	No
	Hungry	Yes	No
	Anxious	Yes	No
	Depressed	Yes	No
	Angry	Yes	No
	To fit in	Yes	No
	Happy	Yes	No
	Sad	Yes	No
	Nervous	Yes	No
	Scared	Yes	No
	Frustrated	Yes	No
	Other	Yes	No

Where

I eat too much	Socialising	Yes	No
	Watching TV	Yes	No
	Cinema	Yes	No
	In a group	Yes	No
	In bed	Yes	No
	While reading	Yes	No
	At work/breaks	Yes	No
	Listening to music	Yes	No
	Other	Yes	No

Why

I eat and snack whenever I need	Love	Yes	No
	Attention	Yes	No
	Security	Yes	No
	I feel important	Yes	No
	To relax	Yes	No
	Reward myself	Yes	No
	Entertainment	Yes	No
	Companionship	Yes	No
	To feel good	Yes	No
	Other	Yes	No

Benefits of healthy eating

The benefits of healthy eating are numerous and remarkable, therefore it is imperative that you understand the benefits of eating healthily and what effect it has on your overall well being. Remember that what you put into your body determines the way you feel, look and function.

Below are some of the benefits of healthy eating;
- o By eating healthy you live longer.
- o You look and feel younger with more increased energy levels.
- o Healthy eating reduces stress.
- o It aids and promotes better sleep.

o Increased physical fitness as you have more energy the your fitness levels increase.

o Healthy eating rejuvenates the mind- a healthy diet is crucial for a healthy mind. Evidence suggests that eating a healthy diet is important to your mental health and that illnesses including depression may be influenced by dietary factors.

o Healthy eating also promotes good skin, eyes, hair and nails.

o By eating healthily you keep illnesses and bay as most of them are caused by a poor diet.

Unhealthy eating related illnesses;

o Coronary Heart Disease: narrowing of the blood vessels that carry oxygen and blood to the heart. People who eat too much fat especially saturated fat are at risk of coronary heart disease, as consuming fat blocks the passageways of blood and oxygen to the heart.

o High Blood Pressure: foods that are high in salt and fats as well as inadequate water in the diet can lead to high blood pressure.

o Type 2 Diabetes: is a disorder in which the blood has too much glucose in it that the body can't process it. Diabetes is often caused by diets that are too high in calories and sugar.

o Cancer: un-healthy eating causes the immune system to be weakened and therefore less prone to fight off certain types of cancers. With a good diet of enough vitamins and nutrients, the immune system has a better chance of fighting off illnesses.

o Obesity: is a medical condition in which excess body fat has accumulated to the extent that it may have a negative impact on health and leading to a reduced life expectancy. According to the National Health Service, obesity is currently a common problem estimated to affect around one in every four adults and around one in every five children aged ten to eleven years in the United Kingdom. Eating foods that are high in sugar and saturated fats leads to obesity. If not tackled obesity can also cause other diseases such as Coronary heart Disease, Type 2 diabetes, some types of cancer like breast and bowel cancer, stroke, depression and also cause low self-esteem and confidence.

o Liver damage- which is common in obese and over weight adults, fat builds up within the liver cells which increases the risks of heart attack and stroke.

o Joint problems due to weight putting a strain on joints especially knee and cartilage tears.

o It affects fertility in both men and women.

o Cholesterol- too much cholesterol leads to it building up in the inner walls of the body's arteries as plaques, as these plaques grow larger and larger the blood vessels' width become narrower until eventually the clot completely cuts off any blood flow through the artery. If the artery leads to the heart, this may cause a heart attack. If the artery leads to the brain then a stroke may occur.

o   Depression and mental illnesses

PLANNING MEALS

A healthy balanced diet should have three meals, a man should need around 2500 calories a day to maintain his weight , where as for a woman it is 2000 calories a day. Although these values vary depending on age, metabolism and levels of physical activity. Healthy eating doesn't have to be expensive, complicated or time consuming!

A healthy balanced diet should include;

o   Plenty of fruit and vegetables - 5 a day
o   Plenty of starchy foods like bread, rice, potatoes, pasta, cassava, yams
o   Some meat, fish, eggs, beans and other diary sources of protein
o   Some milk and dairy foods
o   Good fats
o   Plenty of water
o   Nuts and seeds

Eating planned regular meals not only helps you to eat proper healthy food, but it also helps you to control the amount of food that you eat. And by doing so it prevents you from being hungry and snacking on high calorie snacks. Planning a day's meal should be fun as well as a morale booster.

Breakfast

As we all know breakfast is the most important meal of the day that should not be missed as it kick starts and speeds up your metabolism, helps you feel more energetic and increases your concentration levels. Research suggests that people who eat breakfast are slimmer because they tend to eat less during the day, especially high-calorie snacks. A healthy breakfast should be nutritious, filling and energy-boosting but also high in fibre and low in fat and sugar.

Avoid these foods in the morning;

o Processed foods- bacon, ham, sausages, deep fried eggs
o Sugary cereals
o Pastries- doughnuts, danishes, muffins extra
o Cream and sugar packed coffee drinks
o Bagels, scones, pancakes
o Fizzy drinks
o High sugar smoothies
o Fast food breakfast sandwiches
o Biscuits, cookies
o High sugar orange juice
o Full fat milk with cereal

Lunch

Lunch is an important part of your daily three meals and should be nutritious- full of nutrients to fuel the second half of the day, helps prevent snacking and keeps the metabolism going. Therefore it is vital not to skip lunch to save calories, if you skip lunch you will end up snacking on high calorie foods for energy to keep you going until your dinner meal. If you're trying to lose weight eat a low calorie lunch aiming for 400 to 450 calories and if you're working at maintaining your weight then 500 calories will be ideal.

Dinner

Because dinner is usually the main meal, make it a good one and base it around proteins, complex carbohydrates and vegetables, foods like lean meat, fish, eggs and serve it with rice, pasta, noodles or bread and a selection of vegetables and fruit salad or low fat yogurt for afters. If you eat a good filling meal then you won't feel the urge to dig back into the fridge or cupboard for snacks and nibbles.

Portion Control

Portion control plays a big part in healthy eating, weight loss and maintenance. If you are a big eater you must learn to eat smaller portions. In other words try eating from a smaller plate than a large plate or choose foods that come in ready portions. It is also essential that you don't skip meals, because if you skip meals you are more likely to eat extra large portions. Also add plenty of vegetable to your meal to add volume without adding a lot of calories. And most importantly listen to your hunger cues, stop eating when you're satisfied. Plus if your mind is trained, it will play a big role in controlling how much food you eat and when to stop eating.

Eating out and takeaways

Food is one of life's many pleasures and should be enjoyed whether you go eating out regularly or occasionally. You have to enjoy it without feeling guilty and stressing that you are going to put on weight. The main goal is to keep an eye on what you're ordering and stick to low calorie foods, don't over indulge, and stop eating as soon as you're full. You don't have to finish the food served to you, restaurants are well known for serving large portions and also keep an eye on how much you are drinking as alcoholic drinks stimulate appetite and also add to the calories. And on the other hand if you are ordering a takeaway from home, don't order excess food however tempting it is, stick to keeping the calorie levels as minimum as possible but also enjoy your meal!

Fast food healthy choices

We all eat in fast food restaurants every now and then for instance on days out, at airports, train stations, at work, on holiday and so forth. Eating in restaurants doesn't have be a disastrous fatty food binge resulting in guilt and self-loathing. It is possible to make smart food healthy food choices with a few calories and also be able to enjoy your meal.

Alcohol

Even though drinking is associated with having fun, enjoying and relaxing, it is very easy to get carried away and drink more than necessary. Frequent alcohol consumption is not a healthy habit and can sabotage any weight loss plans for people who want to lose weight. Limiting alcohol consumption helps cut down on the calorie intake as well as maintaining good health. It is a fact that too much alcohol over a long period of time can cause lasting damage to body organs from the liver, heart, lungs, kidneys, brain among others. If you find it impossible to limit your intake then stick to non- alcoholic drinks, you shouldn't have to drink to have a good time. The body metabolizes alcohol in a very different way to how it metabolizes food and other beverages. When you eat food your body breaks it down and uses the calories from carbohydrates, proteins and fat and then digests it within the gastrointestinal system with the nutrients. On the other hand when you drink alcohol your body treats it as toxic and doesn't digest it. Alcohol makes you gain weight in numerous ways;

- o It increases your appetite, alcohol makes you excessively hungry hence you eat more as a result and more often when people drink they crave carbohydrate foods which are high in calories for instance pizza, chips, French fries and other fatty foods.
- o Alcohol slows your metabolism as your body will concentrate on filtering the alcohol in your system and get rid of it rather digesting food.
- o It contains calories - that will go on top of the calories you get from food.

o When you drink alcohol, your body tends to store fat as the food you eat wont be metabolized, it will instead be stored as fat while your body will concentrate on filtering the alcohol.

The effects of alcohol on your body are both mental and physical.

Mental effects;

o It increases stress and anxiety.
o Heavy drinking may cause depression.
o Loss of memory and inability to think clearly as alcohol interferes with the brain's pathways thereby disrupting mood and behaviour.
o Because heavy drinking makes people lose their inhibitions, there is a great risk of suicide and self-harm.

Physical effects;

o Brain- Too much alcohol consumption affects the brain causing blurred vision, difficulty walking, slurred speech, slowed reaction times and impaired memory.
o Heart- drinking too much alcohol over a long period of time or too much on a single occasion can damage your heart causing stroke, high blood pressure, irregular heart beat, cardiomyopathy.
o Liver- too much alcohol damages the liver causing alcohol hepatitis, fatty liver, fibrosis, cirrhosis.
o Pancreas- excess alcohol causes the pancreas to produce excess toxic substances that can subsequently cause

Cancer- drinking excessively can also increase the risk of mouth, esophagus, throat, liver and breast cancers.

o Alcohol in big doses will weaken your immune system making your body susceptible to contacting diseases. It can also lead to alcohol poisoning causing unconsciousness, coma, and even death.

Holidays

When you're trying to stay healthy, lose weight or control it, holidays are a very testing time as people associate them with having fun, indulging and letting go. You can still enjoy your holiday and still keep an eye on your weight and stick to your goals by keeping calories down and not having extras. Eat a good breakfast every day and try and keep your lunches and dinner meals moderate. You can still eat what you want and enjoy it but in smaller portions. Indulging in treats like sweets, ice creams, chocolate and other high calorie treats will make you pile on the pounds , therefore keep your treats at minimum at least once a day. And mostly have plenty of exercise! Just because you are on holiday doesn't mean that you can slop around all day, exercise will do you the world of good, have plenty of walks and get to explore your new surroundings. Likewise go for a jog, run, swimming, tennis, cycling whatever exercise interests you at least once a day. By keeping active you will keep your mind off food and keep it fit and healthy, you will also come back from your holiday feeling relaxed, refreshed, fit and most of all having kept those extra pounds at bay!

Christmas

Whether it is Christmas, birthdays, weddings or any other parties have fun but be sensible. Christmas is the time of the year when most people worry and stress about their weight. The key is to plan it carefully.

When you're out food shopping try and minimise the treats you buy such as sweets, biscuits, chocolates, cakes and alcohol. Remember not to go overboard and go off your healthy eating plan. You can still be sensible but have fun too, buy plenty of healthier Christmas foods and alcohol free wines. The trick is to keep your overall calorie intake to a reasonable level but still have fun. After boxing day its time to get back to your normal eating routine otherwise if you continue to indulge yourself stuffing your neck and face with food you will pile the pounds on.

Healthy snacks- Low in fat and calories

Nuts and Seeds: although nuts are healthy fats, they should be eaten in moderation as they can be high in calories. Ideally rather than eating unhealthy calories, you should substitute them by eating healthy fats from nuts, having a handful or eating them as a spread. These include;

- o Peanuts
- o Almonds
- o Hazel nuts
- o Walnuts
- o Brazil nuts

o Cashew nuts
o Chest nuts
o Sesame seeds
o Sun-flower seeds
o Pumpkin seeds

Fruit and Vegetables: Fruit and vegetables make healthy snacks for instance apples, raisins, grapes, blueberries, raspberries, strawberries, banana, oranges, passion fruit, kiwi, pomegranate, coconut, pears, tangerine, guava, nectarines, plums, pineapple, melon, cherries, papaya, chopped carrots, cucumber, celery, peas, asparagus, cabbage, lettuce, tomatoes, beetroot, peppers.

Foods and drinks to avoid- which are very un-healthy

o Fast foods- chips, burgers, pizza
o Packaged cookies
o Cake
o Popcorn
o Frozen meals
o Fizzy drinks
o High fat yogurt
o Ketchup
o Cereals
o Dressings
o Cheese
o Butter, margarine, lard
o Salty snacks- crisps

o Fatty meats- bacon, beef, pork

o Ice cream, milk shakes, smoothies

o Donuts, bagels, pan cakes,

o Cream

o Coffee drinks

o Chocolate nut spread

o Alcohol

o Oil- highly processed

o Protein bars

o Sweetened condensed milk, whole milk

o Sweets

Healthy eating tips

o Eat a balanced diet and stick to eating three meals a day and avoid skipping any of them as much as you can.

o Eat low fat- calorie foods and control your portions

o Restrict your sugar intake

o Eat plenty of fruit and vegetables

o Restrict your salt intake

o Eat more complex carbohydrates and fibre

o Make sure you're getting enough vitamins and minerals

o Drink plenty of water

o Restrict your alcohol consumption

o Eat whole grain brown pasta, rice, bread

o Monitor your weight at least once a week or a fortnight

o Be positive- your mental well-being is as crucial as your physical well being. The right frame of mind will keep weight off permanently.

o   Don't over-eat

o   Stay motivated and determined not to slip back into your old habits and keep an eye on your weight. If you spot any signs of weight gain for instance if your clothes become tighter then take immediate action, however avoid weighing yourself everyday.

Self-hypnosis script for healthy eating

I will make myself as comfortable as I can ...... take a nice deep breath ...... close my eyes and begin to relax ...... just thinking about relaxing every muscle in my body ..... from the top of my head to the tips of my toes ...... as I begin to focus attention on my breathing ...... my awareness of everything around me will decrease ...... I let all the muscles in my body relax

...... from the top of my head to my toes and as I continue to do this I can feel all the tension and stress leave my mind and body .... I begin to drift into a deeper and deeper relaxation ...... I am feeling lighter and lighter ...... floating higher into an even deeper level of relaxation ..... now that I am completely relaxed ...... more relaxed than I have ever felt before ...... and as I experience this beautiful feeling of peace and calm ...... I just let go of my mind ...... drift ...... relax ....and drift ....

Because I am deeply relaxed now .... I am going to give my subconscious suggestions that it won't be critical of .... suggestions that it will accept and that will help me to eat healthy and stay healthy .... my subconscious mind will accept the new suggestions .... the more and more relaxed I become in my mind and body .... the more the suggestions are going to be effective ...... because my mind is more open to all the positive new thoughts .... feelings .... and attitudes towards food and my goal of eating healthy .... from this day onwards I will have a healthy balanced diet of three meals everyday ...... and I will only chose healthy foods over the unhealthy ones .... now I imagine myself in my favourite supermarket doing my food shopping .... as I enter I take a trolley with me and start to look around ...... at first I am hit by the smell ..... a sweet sugary smell which makes me realise that I am on the isle filled with junk foods ...... and this feeling makes me nauseous ...... and move on to the next isle as quickly as I can ...... this isle is full of colour ...... freshness ...... its the isle of healthy food ...... vegetables ..... fresh fruit ...... fresh bread ...... it's very inviting and the smell fills the air .... I notice that a lot of people in this isle are slim .... and move quickly and easily .... full of strength and life .... full of health ......I fill my trolley with a lot of these nutritious foods ...... and then go through the checkout and head off home to try my healthy food .... at home I prepare myself my right portion of this food and the taste is delicious ...... awakening all my taste buds ......my body feels energised ...... and now I can see the many possibilities of eating healthily ...... as I feel lighter and much more energetic ...... healthy food satisfies my appetite ...... from now on only healthy nutritious foods fill me up and energize me ..... I crave only healthy foods ...... I no longer have the desire to eat un-healthy foods ...... foods high in fat, sugar and salt .... the thought of putting these foods in my mouth again disgusts me .... the thought of eating foods that have a high calorie content appals me ...... junk food no longer smells or tastes good ...... I no longer want to eat big portions of food .... big portions of food are un-healthy for me and make me fat .... I no longer have the need to snack in between meals ...... and when I choose to have a snack I make a healthy choice of fruit, nuts, seeds or munch on vegetables ...... they are the choices for me to keep me healthy ...... and they fill me up and nourish me and that feels just fine .... I drink more water than ever before and keeps me healthy, refreshed and it fills me up ...... water tastes amazing and I find myself drinking more of it everyday ...... my meals are more balanced now and the portions smaller ...... but they still fill me up ...... eating large meals is in the past and will stay in the past ......

Food doesn't control me anymore ...... I control food and when I am full I simply stop eating and leave the excess food on the plate ...... and it feels just fine, easy and natural to me now ...... I treat food with respect because I am in control of my eating habits .... I eat plenty of fruit and vegetables throughout the day everyday and I notice that I feel and look even more healthier ...... my skin is glowing ...... my memory terrific ...... my bones feel stronger ...... and I feel fitter than ever before ..... being healthy suits me perfectly ......

eating is something I do to get energy and live ...... and even find eating healthy food enjoyable .... because when I eat healthy foods I don't feel guilty ...... it rather fills me with happiness and fulfilment that I am giving my body and mind the right food and nutrients it needs to stay healthy ...... and giving my body the best chance of fighting off illnesses and staying fit ...... my mind knows instinctively the right foods for my body ...... from this moment and onwards I will listen more to my gut feeling to make the right choices of food and abandon the un-healthy ones ...... I feel positive and happy ......I am totally in charge of what I choose to eat ...... and I only make healthy choices ...... I am in control ......

I will enjoy this moment of relaxation and calmness for a few more minutes ...... I will continue to relax ..... drift and float ...... I am feeling calm and relaxed ...... and when I am ready to come back to full awareness ......I will count from one to ten .... and as I count from one to ten ...... I will begin to come back to full awareness ...... I will come back feeling at ease and relaxed ....

1.................... Beginning to come back

2.................... The background noises are coming back

3 ....Feeling relaxed

4.................... I am aware of my body

5 ....Feeling calm and peaceful

6 ....I am almost fully alert now

7 ....Feeling relaxed

8 ....I am aware of my normal surroundings

9 ....Beginning to open my eyes now

10 ....I open my eyes and come back feeling wonderful

Healthy eating positive statements

- o I choose to eat only healthy food
- o I make the choice to change my eating habits
- o I love and enjoy eating healthy food
- o I make only choices of healthy food
- o I don't feel the urge to over-eat anymore
- o Small amounts of food fill me up
- o I have a healthy attitude towards food
- o I only eat when I'm hungry and when I'm full I stop eating
- o I eat the right portions of food
- o I have healthy thoughts towards food
- o I treat food with respect
- o I'm healthier and healthier with each day
- o I always eat a balanced diet
- o I have renewed energy and ambition
- o Binge eating is in my past
- o The thought of over-eating does not appeal to me anymore
- o I feel and look better than I've done in ages
- o I eat all three meals every day
- o Eating healthy is becoming part of me and easier
- o I always chose healthy nutritious foods over junk foods
- o Food doesn't control me anymore, I am in control of it now
- o I love my fruit and vegetables
- o I nourish my body with plenty of water

- o Healthy food energizes my body and mind
- o I am a healthy eater and it suits me
- o I eat plenty of fruit and vegetables everyday
- o I eat all vitamins and nutrients that my body needs
- o I feel healthier, fitter and energetic with each day
- o Healthy foods make me healthier
- o My bad eating habits are in the past. I am in charge of what foods I eat now. I only choose healthy foods.

Healthy eating visualization technique

- o Put aside time everyday and practice at least two to three times a day
- o Sit in a quiet place and start by breathing in deeply, let go of the tension in your body and close your eyes ....
- o Visualize yourself in great detail going to the supermarket, at the supermarket you see yourself buying only healthy foods ...... you buy fruit, vegetables, and all the nutritious foods that your body needs to function properly ...... you stay away from all the foods that are high in fat, sugar and salt ...... and you feel fine about it .....
- o By using all your five senses you imagine yourself eating and enjoying every mouthful of the healthy food .... it tastes delicious ..... and smells very nice ..... you feel very energized and a transformation taking place within you ...... you feel happy, healthy and fit ......
- o You now visualize how you want to look like ...... your perfect body and hold on to that mental picture in your mind, see it vividly, how you want to feel and look ...... because you are in the process of creating that ideal body

o Visualize a lot of compliments from your family, friends and work colleagues, visualize all of them admiring the new you, healthy, fit and looking great.

o Continue to visualize yourself eating healthily and sticking with your healthy eating plan and exercise plan ...... you feel great .....

o Hold that image of a healthier and fitter you, you feel so happy and fulfilled because you have achieved your goals and continue to make better choices based on your new healthier image and the knowledge you have acquired. You simply feel and look good exuding tremendous confidence.

o And lastly believe and trust the process without questioning it, I can't reinforce enough that you have to avoid negative thoughts. And be patient and persistent, then you will see the results.

****

Part Three

Weight Loss and the Mind

All weight loss starts in the mind, therefore with our thoughts we can do so much to help improve our body's well being. The body will bring about whatever the mind desires, so your body is always waiting for your command for it to get into action. For instance if you say " I will lose weight" or "I can lose weight" your mind will work towards nothing but aligning all your actions towards getting your body into action to lose weight. By changing the way you think using the power of your mind to eat the right foods in the right amounts, and keeping active you will be on your way to achieving your success with a winning combination which can't be triumphed by any other. Mind power techniques are very powerful to help you develop a new positive relationship with food, change any negative thoughts about eating, make you feel confident about your body and also help you to lose weight in a responsible and healthier way for both the body and mind.

Losing weight is going to be a challenge and any formula that excludes hard is delusional and un-realistic, but one thing I'm certain about is that if you put the hard work in, down the line you will shed the pounds off. The problem is most people want lose weight quick and that's why they opt for quick fixes such as crash diets, diet pills and so forth, unfortunately which are all not the safest ways to lose weight.

Hypnosis is a natural and safe alternative to lose weight with no side effects at all. Self-hypnosis for weight loss will help you to change the way you think and feel about your food choices, by accessing your subconscious mind with effective and powerful suggestion techniques that will help you to develop a healthy and positive relationship with food, change any negative thoughts you have about eating and helping you to lose weight in a more healthier and responsible way without compromising your physical and mental well- being.

WEIGHT LOSS HYPNOSIS SCRIPT

I will make myself as comfortable as I can .... take a nice deep breath ...... close my eyes and begin to relax .... just thinking about relaxing every muscle in my body ...... from the top of my head to the tips of my toes ...... As I begin to focus attention on my breathing ...... my awareness of everything around me will decrease ...... all the muscles in my body are relaxing ...... as I concentrate on breathing in and out .... I am drifting into a deeper and deeper level of relaxation ...... I am feeling lighter and lighter ...... floating higher and higher into a deeper level of relaxation .... I am now completely relaxed ...... more relaxed than I have ever felt before ..... as I experience this beautiful feeling of peace and calm .... I will completely let go of my mind ..... drift, relax and drift ...... my mind is calm, peaceful and relaxed and my whole body is completely and deeply relaxed ......

Now I am imagining myself in my special place ...... I am feeling calm and relaxed here ..... this is a very special place for me ...... I can feel it ...... I am at peace here ...... with no one to disturb me ...... this is my special time ...... my body is relaxing ..... deeper and deeper..... my mind is calm and enjoying these positive feelings .....I am feeling lighter and lighter..... floating into a comfortable relaxation ......

Because I am now at peace and relaxed ...... I accept that I need to lose weight and that I will be successful at reaching my goal of losing weight ..... I will stick to my goal without letting anything or anyone get in the way .... I am going to lose weight and become healthier and thinner ..... beginning right now by relaxing and allowing my subconscious mind to accept all the suggestions ...... I imagine losing the amount of weight that I no longer want and that I will maintain that weight loss ...... I feel and think of myself as slimmer...... and healthier ..... my subconscious will now act on this image and make this image a reality ...... and now I will allow myself to lose weight ..... lose the amount of weight that I longer want and to maintain that weight loss ...... I change my bad eating patterns into good patterns now ..... and choose to become active and exercise everyday to attain my weight loss...... to be a healthy weight starting from now ...... I allow this to take place easily ...... I see myself eating more and more healthy food ...... and I eat modest portions and they fill me up .... feeling completely satisfied ...... and that's fine ..... my whole body feels energised and I see all the many possibilities to eat healthily .... I feel lighter and weigh less with each day ...... and now I imagine seeing myself on my holiday so happy ...... thinner, healthier, stomach flat, hips and thighs firm and trim, legs firm and slim .....

I look great and feel confident and proud of myself and my achievement ..... all my friends think I look wonderful ..... and they are so happy for me ......

Food is less and less important to me ..... and whenever I think of eating I choose those good healthy foods ...... and I eat the correct amount ..... and when I eat the correct amount I stop.

I am more motivated now than ever before to create the most healthy and positive life for myself ..... to change my old bad eating patterns into good new eating patterns ..... to lose the amount of weight I want to lose and to maintain this weight loss ..... I will enjoy being energetic and fit ...... and I will feel more happier, confident and healthier ...... these new habits will make permanent weight loss possible ...... from this moment on ..... I no longer have the urge to over-eat or to snack in between meals .... because healthy, well-balanced meals satisfy my appetite ..... and the taste and fragrance of food are better than ever before ...... I imagine myself exercising everyday ...... burning all those calories my body doesn't need ...... and losing weight quickly and steadily because of all the effort I am putting in .... I lose weight at a steady pace and it keeps falling off ...... with my new fitter and healthy body I find that I have even more energy to exercise more ...... and I put this extra energy to good use by exercising even more .... reaching my ideal weight .... my health increases with each day as I get fitter and fitter ..... all the excess fat on my body is shifting and dropping off .... leaving my body and never to return ...... and that feels wonderful .... I look amazing ...... I feel good and very confident .....

I look very healthy and happy .... this is me and who I want to be ..... and from this day and onwards my past bad habits will stay in the past where they belong ...... I've created new positive changes in my life and that's how its going to be from now and onwards ..... I will eat only healthy foods that nourish my body .... and avoid fatty foods that are high in calories .... From this day and onwards I will exercise regularly to keep my body and mind fit and healthy .... from this moment I will work with my mind and maintain a positive attitude to achieve my dreams and desires. I will continue to enjoy my special place for another moment, experience it ...... drift and float .... I am feeling calm and relaxed ......In a few minutes I will come back to awareness ..... I will count from one to ten and as I count from one to ten I will begin to come back to full awareness .... I will come back feeling calm and relaxed ....

1.................... I am beginning to come back

2.................... All the background noises are coming back again

3 ....I am able to recall the room I'm in

4.................... I am feeling calm and completely relaxed

5 ....I am aware of my whole body

6 ....Feeling calm and peaceful

7 .... I am aware of my surroundings and all the background noises

8 ....Feeling so calm and relaxed

9 ....I am beginning to open my eyes now

10 ....I come back feeling good.

Weight loss positive statements

- I am taking charge to lose weight
- I feel great and I look great.
- I am in control of what I eat.
- I love the foods that keep me healthy.
- I look and feel lighter with each passing day.
- I can feel myself getting fitter and healthier every day.
- I enjoy the process of being healthy and losing weight.
- Everyday I get closer to my ideal weight.
- Maintaining my ideal weight is easy and effortless.
- I enjoy living a healthy and active life.
- I control my weight through regular exercise and what I eat.
- I am fit, attractive and healthy.
- I am the healthiest I have ever been.
- I train my mind to make only healthy choices of food and that feels fine.
- I am extremely confident in myself.
- Losing weight comes naturally to me.
- Being slim and healthy suits me.
- Everyday I get slimmer and healthier.
- I feel great and look great in my clothes as the weight drops off.

o   I am losing all the excess weight.

o   Exercising comes naturally for me and I enjoy it.

o   Exercise is part of my daily routine and keeps me fit.

o   I digest my foods easily by keeping active.

o   I burn a lot of calories with daily exercise.

o   I love my body and take good care of it.

o   I am slimmer, fit and healthy and I will stay slim, fit and healthy.

o   I eat slowly and stop eating the moment I am full

o   I am losing weight slowly and steadily.

o   I enjoy eating small portions of food and drink   lots of water

o   I have eliminated sugar from my food. I now eat only nutritious food.

o   I get a lot of compliments about how fit and healthy I look

o   Healthy eating is a way of life and comes easily to me

o   With each day I lose more and more weight

o   I am attaining and maintaining my ideal weight

o   I will stay fit and healthy by making healthy choices

Weight loss visualization

o   Put aside time everyday and practice at least two to three times a day

o   Sit in a quiet place and start by breathing in deeply, let go of the tension in your body and close your eyes ....

o Visualize yourself in great detail making a choice of only healthy foods when doing your food shopping ...... you see yourself buying only healthy foods ...... you buy fruit, vegetables, and all the nutritious foods that your body needs to function properly ...... you stay away from all the junk foods ...... and you feel fine about it ..... you are not drawn to them anymore because you know that they are not good for your health ...... and they will make you put on weight .....

o By using all your five senses you imagine yourself eating and enjoying every mouthful of the healthy food ...... it tastes delicious ..... and smells very nice ..... you feel very energized and satisfied with every mouthful ..... eliminating any thoughts of fat, weight and dieting ..... you focus on what you want to be and you feel happy because you're transforming your body into that perfect body that you want ..... and most of all you are healthy and fit ......

o You now vividly visualize how you want to look ...... your perfect body......and hold on to that mental picture in your mind, see it vividly, how you want to feel and look ...... because you are in the process of creating that ideal body ...... imagine the weight melting off with each day ..... this is a very powerful process and visualize a lot of compliments from your family, friends and work colleagues, visualize all of them admiring the new you, a healthy, fit person, you look great.

o Continue to visualize yourself eating healthily and
   sticking with your healthy eating plan and exercise plan
   ...... you imagine yourself exercising everyday and the
   more you exercise the more that the weight drops off and
   you can see and feel this taking place you feel great .....

o You hold that image of a healthier and fitter you, you feel
   so happy and fulfilled because you have achieved your
   goals and continue to make better choices based on your
   new healthier image and the knowledge you have
   acquired. You simply feel and look good exhuming
   tremendous confidence.

o You believe and trust the process without questioning it
   because you can feel the transformation already
   happening within you.

Weight loss meditation

1. Begin by focusing your attention on your breathing
   going deeply within with each breath let yourself go
   deeper and deeper into a beautiful, relaxed and
   tranquil state.

2. Focus on your breathing and as you do this relax all
   your muscles and feel yourself going even deeper, take
   note of those thoughts going through your mind and
   let them go as they come.

3. As you let go of all the tension and stress in your body
   you relax even more, now visualize a beautiful white
   light coming in through the top of your body from

above to below entering your brain and going through every part of your body, glowing, healing, protecting and relaxing you even deeper.

4. Now you feel very calm, peaceful and relaxed, you continue to focus on your breathing and try as much as possible to clear your mind letting go of all the chatter of thoughts running through it, don't judge or analyse anything, you are only observing.

5. Now in this relaxation, visualize an image of yourself eating healthily, exercising everyday with a positive mind, see yourself looking healthy and fit ..... your ideal weight, you look good and feel good about yourself. You can also focus on a word or mantra if its easier for you something like "healthy", "fit", "slim" whatever feels right for you is fine, say it mentally again and again and if any negative thoughts pop up try and replace them with happy positive ones and bring your attention back to your breathing.

6. Continue holding the image or mantra as long as you can.

Weight loss relaxation

Relaxation technique is suitable for people who suffer from emotional eating and stress, as research has found that by learning and practicing relaxation you can manage stress without turning to un-healthy eating. When the body is under stress, it creates more fat and less glycogen so when you reduce stress you will reduce weight. Relaxation is helpful in way that you are able to let go of tension in your body and mind.

Like all the other mind techniques, relaxation will require a lot of practice and persistence for it to be an effective tool for weight loss.

Weight loss relaxation technique

Close your eyes and sit back comfortably with your feet together .... hands resting on the sides of the chair or on your thighs .... take a nice deep breath and begin to relax ..... breath in again and hold your breath ...... then let go of it and feel yourself letting go of all the stress and tension as you breath out ...... just think about relaxing every muscle in your body from your head to your toes ...... and keep breathing deeply in and out ...... feeling the calm and relaxation flowing through your body relaxing you all over .... every time you breath out you become more and more completely relaxed ...... now think about nothing else but how your body feels ..... continuing to breath in and out ...... now focus on the muscles around your eyes and around your mouth ...... let them relax ...... and the muscles in your jaw are completely relaxed too .....feel them relax even more as you drift and float into a deeper level of relaxation ...... let the muscles in your neck and shoulders relax ...... filling you with soothing relaxation .... the relaxation spreads to muscles in your back ...... running down your arms and your finger tips as you continue to breath in and out feeling completely relaxed .... now I want you to notice this same feeling moving to your chest, stomach and thighs ...... you breath in and relax these muscles and as you breath out you relax the muscles in your legs .... to the tips of your toes .... your whole body is covered with a complete sense of relaxation ..... you are floating deeper .... and deeper ....

Now count from one to five and as you count from one to five ...... you will let yourself sink more and more deeply into this nice relaxed state ...... One ..... deeper and deeper ...... Two ...... you feel more and more relaxed ..... Three ..... you are sinking deeper and deeper ...... Four ...... you feel so heavy and relaxed ..... Five ...... you feel even more relaxed with every breath ......

Now that you're so deeply relaxed ...... imagine yourself in your special place ...... a place that means a lot to you and makes you feel loved, happy, calm and at peace ...... whilst in this calm and deeply relaxed state you think about your weight loss goals ...... and how you are going to achieve them ...... you formulate a plan in your head calm and relaxed ..... you see yourself succeed with all your plans and that feels amazing ..... you enjoy these tranquil positive feelings and keep them with you ...... you allow these feelings to grow stronger and stronger and spread through all your body and mind ..... you feel good inside and out in this place ...... with a sense of tremendous well-being surrounding you ...... and these positive feelings will remain with you for a long time ...... you calmly breathe in and out and continue to experience this deep state of relaxation which flows through all your body ......

You can remain in this relaxed state as long as you wish ......
when you're ready you will count from one to five ...... slowly
feeling your body returning to its normal state ...... and your
mind becoming more alert ...... on the count of five you will
open your eyes and you will feel relaxed, calm and at peace ......

****

Part Four

Weight Control and the Mind

The trick and secret of maintaining a healthy weight and staying slim is to have the right mindset that will sustain you for the long term. As you know that the root of your actions stems directly from your mind, to be able to stick to your healthy eating plan of a nutritious balanced diet and your daily exercise plan to manage your weight, you will have to get your mind firmly focussed to do that. If you are eating more than you need and exercise very little or none at all and don't have the right positive attitude, then that's why you are piling the weight you had lost back on and struggling to maintain your desired weight. You should avoid making the same mistake again. And if by chance the weight starts to creep back on, then you should resolve to do something about it immediately. Weight loss management can be challenging but also important, as by maintaining a healthy weight you reduce the future risks of weight related illnesses and early death.

Keeping a positive healthy eating and exercise will also benefit your overall health and weight control. Hence keeping weight off is about re-programming new ways of thinking, developing new habits, attitudes and behaviours. Not forgetting motivation which is a very important key to successful weight loss control as it pushes you to achieve your goals because it's engineered by ambition and desire.

Weight control self-hypnosis

Hypnosis is one of the powerful weight control methods there is, by using the power of suggestion, because its very powerful, hypnosis will help you to highlight, accept and emphasise a positive thinking mind, healthy eating habits and exercising. The subconscious mind transforms habits into healthy patterns which are designed to help you make those changes that you need to make and put you back in control so that you can achieve your goal of maintaining a healthy weight. The reasons why you are over-eating or averse to exercise are embedded in your mind and that's where the work has to begin to change the way you think, feel and behave around food.

Weight control self-hypnosis script

I will make myself as comfortable as I can .... take a nice deep breath ...... close my eyes and begin to relax .... just thinking about relaxing every muscle in my body ...... from the top of my head to the tips of my toes ......

As I begin to focus attention on my breathing ...... my awareness of everything around me will start to fade away ...... and as everything fades away I feel more and more relaxed ...... all the muscles in my body are relaxing ...... as I concentrate on breathing in and out .... I am drifting into a deeper and deeper level of relaxation ...... I am becoming more and more relaxed with every breath I take ...... I drift into a deeper level of relaxation .... I am now completely relaxed ...... more relaxed than I have ever felt before ..... as I experience this beautiful feeling of peace and calm .... I completely let go of my mind ..... drift and relax ...... my mind is calm, peaceful and relaxed and my whole body is completely and deeply relaxed ...... more relaxed than I have ever been before .... completely relaxed ......Now I am imagining myself in my special place ...... I am feeling calm and relaxed here ..... this is a very special place for me ...... I can feel it ...... I am at peace here ...... there is no one to disturb me ..... or demand my attention ...... this is my special time ...... for my body and mind to relax ...... my body is relaxing ..... deeper and deeper..... my mind is calm and enjoying these positive feelings .....I am feeling lighter and lighter..... floating into a comfortable relaxation ......

Because I am now completely relaxed and at peace ...... I can be successful at reaching my goal of managing my weight .... maintaining my perfect weight .... because it was easy for me to lose all the extra weight I needed to lose ...... it is going to be even easier for me to maintain my weight and stay a healthy weight ...... it's been months since I binge ate or had any junk food cravings ...... and I haven't missed it one single bit ...... because I am a stronger person now ...... and find it easy to stay in control of what I eat and in what amounts ...... I find it easy to stick to my exercise routine and it works for me .... I feel better in my life than I have ever felt before ...... I look and feel good about myself ...... I have more energy .... I am healthy ...... toned ...... and fit ...... and my self-confidence is better than before .....I no longer feel the need to eat foods packed with fat, sugar and salt

...... I only crave and choose healthy nutritious food ...... because I am in complete control of my body, mind and well-being .... I am becoming healthier and thinner with each day ...... and now that I am more relaxed than ever before my subconscious mind will accept all the suggestions ......

And now, I am imagining maintaining a healthy weight ..... my ideal perfect weight ...... my perfect body ...... flat stomach ...... tighter skin ...... toned body ...... because having a healthy and fit body is very important to me ...... and its a great feeling .... I think of myself as slimmer, fitter and healthier ..... and from now on my subconscious will act on this image and make this image a reality ...... and I will allow myself to control my weight ..... I will work positively with my mind to stick to my healthy eating plan ..... and to exercise everyday ..... I choose to become active and exercise everyday to attain my ideal weight ...... to be a healthy weight starting from now ...... I allow this to take place easily ...... I imagine myself working out everyday and enjoying how I feel so energized and uplifted after working out ...... burning all the calories and fat that my body doesn't need ...... and I know I am getting in shape with everyday I do this .... this is a great routine for me and it's working out for me ...... it's a successful way for keeping me healthy and in shape ...... I am in the best shape of my life and all my favourite clothes look nice on me ...... exercising nourishes my body and mind ...... in fact I feel more healthier with each exercise .... mentally strong ...... physically strong .... I love exercise because it allows me to create my body ...... to design my body the way I want it to look ......

Now I imagine all those healthy foods .... the foods that fuel my body with the energy I need to function .... and now I can imagine eating all these healthy foods .... and I eat slowly and slowly .... I am aware of the amount of food I am eating ...... and I eat small portions and then stop when I am full ..... I simply stop and that feels just fine .... I find that even with small portions food I have eaten I feel completely satisfied ...... my whole body feels energised and nourished ...... I see all the benefits to eating healthily ...... I am healthy ..... fitter ..... and I look great and feel good about myself ..... all my friends think I look fantastic ..... and they are so happy for me ...... which motivates me even more to stay on track ...... I have a good relationship with food now ..... I see it as a fuel for my body to function ...... and something I can enjoy in the right amounts without feeling guilty ...... and whenever I think of eating I choose those good healthy foods ...... and I eat the correct amount ..... and when I am full I stop eating and relax ...... and because I am more motivated now than ever before to create the most healthy and positive life for myself ..... and to control my weight.

...... I am determined that these new habits will make permanent weight management possible for me...... because from this moment on ..... I no longer have the urge to overeat or to snack in between meals .... because healthy well-balanced meals satisfy my appetite completely ..... and the taste and fragrance of healthy food is better than that of junk food filled with empty calories ...... and if I choose to snack in between meals I will choose only healthy snacks ...... I will chose fruit ...... vegetable sticks ...... un-salted nuts and other healthy snacks .... I feel very healthy, positive and happy .... this is me and who I want to be ..... I feel a sense of empowerment and achievement .... and this makes me extremely proud of myself ..... achieving my goal of maintaining a healthy weight and ...... I am in complete control of life and well-being and this is how I will continue into the future ......I will remain in this relaxed, calm and peaceful state for another couple of minutes to enjoy these wonderful and positive feelings ...... enjoy being here in my special place knowing that I can always come back here and enjoy these feelings whenever I wish ...... I will continue to drift and float ...... I am feeling completely calm and relaxed ...... In a few minutes I will come back to awareness ..... I will count from one to ten and as count from one to ten I will begin to come back to full awareness .... I will come back feeling calm and relaxed .....

1....................I am beginning to come back

2....................All the background noises are coming back again

3 ....I am able to recall the room I'm in

4....................I am feeling calm and completely relaxed

5 ....I am aware of my whole body

6 ....Feeling calm and peaceful

7 ....I am aware of your surroundings and all the background noises

8 ....Feeling so calm and relaxed

9 ....I am beginning to open my eyes now

10 .... I come back feeling completely relaxed

Weight control positive statements

- o I am on track with my weight control plan.
- o I let go of all my bad eating habits.
- o My body responds to my new way of eating.
- o My body responds to my healthy eating diet.
- o I feel better in my clothes ever than before.
- o I am what I think and eat.
- o I am slimmer, fit and healthy.
- o I am in the best shape of my life.
- o I let go of all my negative thoughts towards food.
- o I let go of all my negative thinking towards exercise.
- o I exercise daily without fail.
- o Exercise is part of my life now.
- o Exercise enables me to maintain my ideal weight.
- o I am making all the right choices to maintain a healthy weight.
- o I am attaining and maintaining my perfect weight.
- o I am strong and healthy.
- o I take good care of my body.
- o I am finding it easy to manage my weight.
- o I am becoming more and more disciplined and focussed with each day.

o I am finding it easy to stay in shape.

o Weight control is my priority and I stick to it.

o I keep a positive attitude about my goals.

o I overcome any challenges that come my way with confidence.

o I am in complete control of my well being.

o I am committed to maintaining my perfect weight.

o Staying healthy makes me feel and look great.

o I am successful with my weight control.

o I am staying away from diets that are not realistic and healthy.

o I maintain my weight with a positive frame of mind.

o I believe in my abilities to stay on track.

o I am at peace with my weight and shape.

o My body is stronger, fitter and healthier.

o I love and accept myself for who I am.

o I am motivated to keep a positive mind, eat healthy, and exercise daily to maintain my ideal weight and I am succeeding at it.

Weight control visualization

o Put aside time everyday and practice at least two to three times a day

o Sit in a quiet place and start by breathing in deeply, let go of the tension in your body and close your eyes ....

o Visualize yourself in great detail making a choice of only healthy foods when doing your food shopping ...... you see yourself buying only healthy foods ...... you buy fruit, vegetables, and all the nutritious foods that your body needs to function properly ...... you stay away from all the junk foods ...... and you feel fine about it ..... you are not drawn to them anymore because you know that they are not good for your health ...... and they will make you put on weight .....

o By using all your five senses you imagine yourself eating and enjoying every mouthful of the healthy food ...... it tastes delicious ..... and smells very nice ..... you feel very energized and satisfied with every mouthful ..... eliminating any thoughts of fat, weight and dieting ..... you focus on what you want to be and you feel happy because you're transforming your body into that perfect body that you want ..... and most of all you are healthy and fit ......

o You now vividly visualize how you want to look ...... your perfect body.... and hold on to that mental picture in your mind, see it vividly, how you want to feel and look ...... because you are in the process of creating that ideal body ...... imagine the weight melting off with each day ..... because this is a very powerful process and it is working right now ......

o Visualize a lot of compliments from your family, friends and work colleagues, visualize all of them admiring the new you, a healthy, fit and you look great.

o Continue to visualize yourself eating healthily and sticking with your healthy eating plan and exercise plan

105

...... you imagine yourself exercising everyday and the more you exercise the more that the weight drops off and you can see and feel this taking place.....you feel more in control with the food choices you make ..... and how much you eat ...... and it feels fine ..... because you're in the process of managing your weight .... and you can see its working for you ...... you're doing just fine ......

o You hold that image of a healthier and fitter you, you feel so happy and fulfilled because you are getting to where you want to be with each day ...... as you continue to make those better choices based on your new healthy lifestyle ...... and the knowledge you have acquired ..... you feel in total control of sculpting your body shape how you want it to be ...... right now ...... and that feels amazing ....

o As you continue experiencing these wonderful feelings you ..... believe and trust that all this is taking place right now because you can feel the transformation already happening within you ......

Tips for weight loss maintenance motivation

o Accept that you have a problem and make a decision that you are going to lose weight and stay healthy, don't over-analyse the problem and give excuses, these will only create doubts and confusion then defeat. You have to find the strength to say "I am going to do this" and NOW. As the power is in the NOW.

106

o Set yourself a goal as this will make it easier for you to motivate yourself to lose weight and keep it off. But its important that you are realistic with your goals, make sure they are achievable. Goals will keep you motivated and moving into the right direction, you can write them down and stick them where you can see them everyday like on your fridge, bedside cabinet, work desk and so forth.

o Be persistent and patient as there will always be set backs, but don't give up sometimes you have to work extra hard to achieve success.

o A positive mind-set will take you a long way- think yourself healthy, fit and slim.

o Set yourself a deadline and stick with it, this will make you work even harder and stay focussed to achieve your goal in your time frame.

o Socialise with people who inspire you to lose weight and keep you motivated. In other words avoid people who practice bad eating habits and influence you to be the same. They will set you back!

o And lastly reward yourself for your hard work as this provides an incentive to keep going, for example you can buy yourself a new outfit to go with your new look!

NOTE: Don't forget, weight management should be looked at as a long-term behavioural change rather than a short-term strategy.

****

Part Five

EXERCISE AND THE MIND

Exercise is activity requiring physical effort which results in a healthier level of physical and mental fitness and strength. There is clearly no weight-loss program or regime that will yield any results without exercise. Exercise burns calories, builds muscle and is vital for increasing the metabolism and by doing so you burn more calories and lose weight. Once you get into the routine of exercising everyday you will enjoy it and feel down when you miss a day! Exercise can reduce your risk of major illnesses such as heart disease, stroke, diabetes and some cancers by 50% and lower your risk of early death by up to 30%.

More so, your mind is the most powerful tool for maintaining an active lifestyle and attitude. If you can win the biggest battle of training your mind, then you can achieve anything! You have to work with your mind so that it can help you remove the blockages, fear and negative thoughts you associate with exercise and keeping fit. When you fill your mind with healthy thoughts, then you will give it a kick up the bum to produce good health and your actions will be geared towards a healthy lifestyle, hence exercising regularly. You have to affirm to yourself that you're fit and healthy, be positive and don't give up at the first hurdle or at all. Believe in your inner strength it will take you a long way and you will be immensely surprised by the success of your hard work.

The health benefits of exercise

According to the National health Service (NHS) it is medically proven that people who exercise regularly have;

o Up to 35 % lower risk of coronary heart disease and stroke.

o Up to 50% lower risk of type 2 diabetes

o Up to 50% lower risk of colon cancer

o Up to 20% lower risk of breast cancer

o Up to 30% lower risk of early death

o Up to 35% lower risk of osteoarthritis

o Up to 68% lower risk of hip fracture

o Up to 30% lower risk of falls (among older patients)

o Up to 30% lower risk of depression

o Up to 30% lower risk of dementia

Other benefits of exercise are;

o When you engage in physical activity, you burn more calories, the more activity the more calories you burn.

o Exercise improves moods as physical activity stimulates numerous brain chemicals that induce feelings of happiness and relaxation.

o Regular exercise improves your muscle strength and boosts endurance, activity delivers oxygen and nutrients to your tissues and helps your cardiovascular system work more efficiently and thereby boosting your energy levels.

o Exercise promotes a better sleeping pattern.

o It improves digestion.

o Regular exercise can reduce high blood pressure and lower levels of bad cholesterol.

o Exercise relieves stress and anxiety and depression.

o It sets a good example to children and will encourage them to stay active and prevent them from becoming obese.

o It's free, easy and has immediate effects on both body and mind health.

Types of exercise

Aerobic exercise: Also known as cardio, this is physical exercise of low/high intensity, it requires pumping of oxygenated blood by the heart to deliver oxygen to working muscles. Aerobic exercise stimulates the heart and breathing rate in a way that can be sustained for the exercise or activity session. Aerobic exercise has immense benefits in keeping fit, losing weight and maintaining weight.

Benefits of aerobic exercise

o It increases energy levels

o Reduces stress, depression and anxiety

o Increases heart and lung efficiency

o Reduces blood pressure rate, heart rate, risk of stroke or heart attack

Examples of aerobic exercises are;

o Running
o Walking
o Swimming
o Cycling
o Rowing
o Aquarobics
o Boxing
o Dancing
o Hiking
o Tennis
o Kick boxing
o Football
o Kayaking
o Basketball
o Volleyball
o Netball
o Skipping
o Trampolining
o Gymnastics

Walking- Walking is a great way to improve and maintain your overall weight. It's free and easy and doesn't have to be strenuous and should be done at your own pace at least thirty minutes or more most days of the week. An energetic walk can burn up to one hundred and ninety five calories (195) in thirty minutes. Walking is a suitable exercise for everyone, young, old, expectant mothers and those who are unable to take part in other sports. In cases of obesity walking would be the perfect starting point as it will help you drop the excess pounds safely without putting too much strain on your heart, joints or muscles. It is advisable that you start off slowly and then increase your pace as your body gets used to it and the weight will start to fall off.

Walking is also a perfect way of exercising in pregnancy although gently, it increases energy levels, boosts circulation, reduces stress, backache, constipation, tiredness and swelling and improves sleep. It is also an ideal exercise for people over 50 as it helps keep bones strong, keep the heart healthy and also keeping depression at bay. The benefits of walking are that;

- o It increases cardiovascular and pulmonary fitness(heart and lung)
- o You burn fat while walking
- o It reduces risk of heart disease and stroke
- o Joint and muscular pain are reduced
- o Stronger bones and improved balance
- o Lowers risk of diabetes
- o Increases muscle strength and endurance

Walking tips

- o Walk to work, to the shops, train, bus stop
- o Walk the kids to school if its a short journey
- o Use the stairs rather than the lift
- o Make sure you have the right pair of shoes that provide comfort and adequate support.
- o Wear loose fitting clothing that you feel comfortable in

o Aim for at least thirty minutes or more but any exercise is better than no exercise!

Running- Running is another great way to keep in shape and as well as benefiting the body, it lifts your moods and it's free. Research shows that running can raise your levels of cholesterol while also helping you increase lung function use. The benefits of running are;

o It improves heart and bone health
o Burns calories at a greater rate
o Better cardiovascular fitness
o Stronger leg muscles
o Relieves stress
o Eliminates depression
o Better sleep
o Boosts confidence

Running tips

o The perfect technique when it comes to running is to do whatever feels natural and comfortable for you, there is no one fit for everyone!
o Get the right pair of shoes- keep in mind that when you run your feet hit the ground with a force up to four times your body weight. So in order to prevent injuries you need a good pair of running shoes, they don't have to be expensive, but comfortable.

- o The clothing has to be comfortable too, either jogging pants or shorts depending on the weather, the socks must also be put into consideration, they should be comfortable and clean, avoid dirty socks to prevent athletes foot!
- o If you are looking to lose weight quickly running is the best exercise as it burns more calories and fat per minute than the other exercises. It burns two and a half times more calories in half an hour than walking does.
- o When you're running water is essential, you have to keep your body hydrated as much as possible before, during and after running.

Swimming- Swimming is an excellent way of keeping fit and also helping to lose weight and maintain it. Swimming works all your body muscles and therefore will help you tone up as well as slim you down. Swimming also burns a lot of calories and has lots of cardiovascular health benefits. Regular swimming will improve your health and may reduce the risk of heart disease as your heart and lungs get stronger. It will also lower the risk of diabetes, stroke and high blood pressure. The benefits of swimming are;

- o It burns fat
- o Improves strength and builds muscle
- o Improves flexibility in the muscles and joints
- o Aids quick recovery from injury
- o It relaxes the body and mind
- o Relieves stress

Cycling- Cycling is a healthy exercise which if done regularly can improve your physical and mental health. Cycling is also a good way to keep fit, lose weight and manage it as it raises your metabolic rate, builds muscle and burns body fat fast. Cycling burns up to 1200 kilojoules (around 300 calories) per hour. The health benefits of cycling are;

o It increases cardiovascular fitness
o Increased muscle strength and flexibility
o Improved joint mobility
o Improved posture and co-ordination
o It strengthens the bones
o Burns fat
o Reduces stress, depression and anxiety

Yoga-is one of the mind-body exercises which can be helpful with flexibility, strength, reduce stress, lower high blood pressure, improve sleep and weight loss and control. Yoga is a good exercise for people who don't like outdoor exercise or going to the gym. Yoga is great with the mind too and can change the way you think therefore a useful tool in rehabilitating your exercising and eating habits.

Pilates- Pilates is an exercise that focuses on mind and body, muscle strength, tone and total body workout which will help with weight loss by increasing muscle tone and therefore the more calories you burn. Pilates can be practiced by people of all ages.

Anaerobic exercise- Anaerobic exercise is a short lasting high intensity activity where your body's demand of oxygen exceeds the oxygen supply available. Anaerobic exercise requires a huge amount of energy and burns fewer calories than aerobic exercise and may not have a big impact on weight loss although it builds and strengthens the muscles and joints and also benefits the heart and the lungs.

Examples of anaerobic exercises are;

o Weight lifting
o Sprinting- running, cycling
o Jumping
o Squats
o Push ups
o Lunges
o Hill climbing
o Jumping rope
o Isometrics

Health benefits of aerobic exercise are;

o It builds and maintains muscle
o It protects joints-increasing muscle strength and mass and helps protect joints- protecting you from injury
o Anaerobic exercise boosts metabolism
o It increases bone strength and density
o Improves your energy levels
o Increases sports performance- strength, speed and power

Metabolism and Exercise

When you exercise, your body requires more energy and your metabolism speeds up to supply it. The more active you are, the more calories you will burn. It's a fact that everyone will lose weight when they burn more calories than they eat. Exercise on a daily basis is going to have an impact on not only your body weight but also your metabolic rate which is what will help you to lose weight and control it as well. This goes to show what a tremendous role exercise plays in weight control. Never-the-less, there is a vast amount of evidence that suggests that diets are doomed to failure, Numerous studies have looked at dieting and diet types and have concluded that attempts at weight loss in that manner are largely un-successful, even in highly controlled situations.

Exercise and longevity

Exercise is associated with a longer life expectancy even when done at relatively low levels, although the benefits increase as you gradually increase your activity levels. Exercise lowers blood pressure, reduces the risk of heart attack and stroke, reduces obesity and lowers the risks of certain cancers and boosts mental health. In summary, exercise extends life expectancy by decreasing the risk of a variety of different ailments and conditions.

Exercise and mental health

Research suggests that exercise provides serious mental health benefits regardless of age. Exercise is one of the easiest and most effective ways to improve mental health. When you exercise the brain releases chemicals that make you feel good, boosting and uplifting your moods and also helping with self-esteem and confidence.

Health benefits of exercise to mental health

o Regular exercise helps keep depression at a distance
o Exercise is a very effective stress management technique, it realises all the negative energies that stress creates and stores in the body.
o It prevents cognitive mental decline, it boosts the chemicals in the brain that support and prevent degeneration of that part of the brain that is responsible for memory and learning.
o It also reduces anxiety and takes your mind off your worries and calms you down.
o Exercise improves self-confidence and esteem.
o It is helpful in addiction recovery by distracting addicts from their addiction and making them divert their cravings to exercise.
o Increases relaxation and positivity
o Aids better sleep

Exercise and weight loss

Losing weight requires a great deal of mental and physical strength and also dedication. Weight is lost by creating calorie deficit, burning more calories than you consume, therefore taking part in exercises that burn large amounts of calories is an excellent way of shedding off all the excess pounds you want to lose. The most effective way to boost your metabolism is by exercising which enables you to burn more calories, the more active you are the more calories you burn. It won't happen over night but if you stick to it, it will guarantee long- lasting results.

Exercise and weight maintenance

Well you've come along way and you have lost all the weight you wanted to lose, well done! But remember that you have to control your weight so that you don't slip back to your old habits of no or less activity, and don't be tempted either to keep eating healthily but stop exercising regularly, you have to stay active to stay on the wagon. This will still require effort and commitment to keep that weight off. Aerobic exercises like running, walking, swimming and cycling are great with weight maintenance.

Reasons why people don't exercise

o Lack of time-with work, children and the other commitments of daily life. In this case you have to set time aside to exercise, even if its only 10 to 20 minutes of exercise it's better than none at all.

119

o Overweight or obesity-people who are overweight or obese generally find it hard to exercise because of the excess weight they are carrying around restricts movement and causes restlessness, nevertheless you should try and start exercising at a very slow pace and then increase with time when the weight starts to drop off and believe me it will if you stick to it and don't give up. Sitting around doing nothing will achieve nothing but worsen your situation. You have more to gain than lose.

o Slim- being slim doesn't guarantee fitness. The fact is that if you're not exercising you're not getting the physical and mental benefits of exercise.

o Boring-there are number of people who don't exercise because they think that exercise is boring. The trick is to find an activity that you enjoy and try and switch things every now and then so that you don't get into that tedious routine that will put you off your activity.

o Age-You are never too old to exercise as exercise benefits people from all different age groups, in fact in older people exercise can increase strength, stability, flexibility and other age related conditions like arthritis, osteoporosis, hypertension and diabetes. With daily exercise these can all be kept at bay.

o Too tired- we all have busy lives and are too tired after a long days of work but exercise will do wonders even if it's only a quick walk, you will feel uplifted, more energized and stress free.

o Not having time off from the children- if this is the case take the children with you for a walk, jog, swim, cycling or any other activity you will all enjoy doing together if you cant venture outdoors then games like wii sport, wii fit and fitness dvds can be helpful in getting you all working out in the comfort of your own home. Also exercises like yoga and pilates can be done from home.

o Hate exercise- there are many forms of exercises and activities that you can take part in if you hate the outdoors. Exercise indoors, walk up and down the stairs, get in some fun fitness dvds that you can borrow from the library, wii sport, wii fit, if you have a dog take it for a walk.

o Lack of motivation- you will have to draw yourself an exercise plan or diary and set yourself targets. If you find it hard to motivate yourself then join a group of people who share your interests and keep with whatever activity you chose to do as the more you do it the more you get into it.

o Laziness- some people are just too lazy to get off their couches to exercise. There is no excuse for that so do yourself a favour and get moving and start reaping all the health benefits of exercising that you're missing out on.

Tips on keeping active and maintaining an active lifestyle

o Start off slowly but keep it steady and constant and build it up gradually.

- o Make small changes in your routine to keep it fresh and exciting, avoid doing the same activity day in day out as this will become monotonous and put you off.
- o Set yourself goals which are realistic and achievable- start off small and then increase as you achieve them.
- o Join a group for moral support if you find it hard to self-motivate, it could be your friends or family who are interested in the same activity as you.
- o Be persistent and don't give up, stick to your goals.
- o With every achievement or milestone you make reward yourself, this will fuel your desire to achieve your goal even more and feel a sense accomplishment and being in control.

Exercise diary

Day exercised	Type of exercise	Length of time
Monday		
Tuesday		
Wednesday		
Thursday		
Friday		
Saturday		
Sunday		

You know now that the mind controls your thoughts, behaviours, attitudes and beliefs. Everything starts in the mind as does the motivation to exercise. Self-hypnosis will help you to re-programme your mind from not wanting to exercise or disliking exercise to liking exercising and actually enjoy doing it on a regular basis. Hypnosis will also benefit you in the following ways;

- o Relaxation
- o Positive mental attitude
- o Mental strength
- o Improve your confidence
- o Overcome mental blocks
- o Visualize success
- o Change the way you think about exercise

Exercise motivation self-hypnosis script

I will make myself as comfortable as I can ...... take a nice deep breath ..... close my eyes and begin to relax ..... I will just think about relaxing every muscle in my body ...... from the top of my head to the tips of my toes .....

As I begin to focus attention on my breathing .... my awareness of everything around me will decrease .... I will let all the muscles in my body relax ..... I will concentrate on relaxing every muscle in my body and my breathing .... relaxing completely .... I notice the rate of my breathing slowing down ...... and every time I breath in and out I relax even more and more ...... I now I am beginning to let go of all the tension in my body .... and relaxing my entire body even more ...... I am drifting deeper and deeper into a comfortable relaxation .... I feel lighter and lighter .... floating higher and higher .... I am completely relaxed .... more relaxed than I have ever felt before .... as I experience this beautiful feeling of peace and calm ...... I let go of my mind ...... drifting ....relaxing .... and drifting ...... feeling completely at ease and relaxed ......

Now that I am deeply relaxed and feeling safe .... I imagine being in my special place ...... a place where I can completely relax and let go of my worries and stresses .... a place for me to relax ...... just me .... in this place I feel safe ..... calm and protected ...... its serene .... I can see it vividly ...... and feel its tranquil and warmth ...... I am feeling my body even relax more here .... no one wants anything from me here .... its my time .... its all about me .... no stress ...... no fear ...... no worries .... anxiety .... its total peace and bliss .... as I enjoy these positive feelings .... I am feeling lighter and lighter .... floating higher and higher into a comfortable relaxation ...... feeling wonderful inside and out ....

Now that I am at peace and relaxed in my special place ......I make a decision ...... an important decision that will make a positive impact on my life ...... the decision to be active everyday ...... the decision to exercise regularly .... this is the right decision for me because it will help me stay healthy ...... it will help me to lose all the weight I want to lose ...... it will help me to maintain a healthy weight .... by exercising regularly I will stay healthy and fit ...... its the right decision for me and I will find it easy to stick to my exercise routine ...... with the help of my subconscious mind .... with the full support of that deeper part of my mind to .... eliminate all my bad habits of laziness and not wanting to exercise .... all the unsettled emotions and feelings I had about exercising .... feelings of discomfort and anxiety .... feelings of panic .... feelings of fear .... and all the wrong assumptions about keeping active which have been holding me back and unsettling me ....from now on ..... I am setting myself free from all those fears and wrong assumptions .... they are not useful to me .... they are destructive to my health and well-being .... and therefore not desirable or appropriate .... they are frightening .... and setting me back from achieving my goals ....

And as I relax even deeper and deeper ...... I begin to realise that I love to exercise and the way I feel when I am exercising and when I finish exercising .... it feels so good and relaxing ...... I love everything about exercising ...... it has so many health benefits .... it's good for my body and my mind .... and with each work out I burn calories which helps me to lose weight and get fitter and healthier .... Now I imagine myself exercising .... I am relaxed and having fun and I can feel my body become more and more energetic .... I am focussed on getting the perfect health ...... the perfect and fit body that I desire .... keeping active will help me design my ideal body .... and nothing is going to stop me achieving it ...... if I encounter any obstacles I will simply view them as challenges .... challenges that I will have to overcome to attain my goal .... I am more focussed than I have ever been before and it feels right ...... I have made one of the best decisions of my life ...... my body and mind feel nourished and renewed after exercising ...... and it feels fine ......

wonderful ...... I no longer make excuses to get active ...... because I have no excuses anymore ...... I simply love exercising and enjoy it everyday ...... its become part of my routine and my life ...... and that is how it is going to be from now on....... my anxious thoughts about exercising are in the past ...... all blown away like the wind .... I am feeling stronger and stronger ...... more and more confident .... and more in control .... I have nothing to fear ..... I am now able to cope ...... and stick to my plan ...... because I am more capable now than ever before .... will the help of my subconscious mind .... I am in charge of my thoughts, feelings and emotions ...... I think positive ...... which in return gives me an overall positive feeling and strength to achieve my goals .... with confidence .... this is the new me ..... fitter ..... healthier ...... and slimmer .... from now and onwards ....

I will enjoy my special place for a few more moments ...... floating and drifting into a deeper relaxation with every breath .... enjoying the positive feelings and calmness .... and then I will come back to full consciousness feeling stronger and more positive .... feeling confident and strong .... in a moment I will count from one to ten and with each number I will become more and more awake .... with beautiful feelings flowing through my body .... calm and peaceful thoughts going through my mind ...... I will wake up feeling fine .... feeling calm .... peaceful .... confident ....

1 .... I am beginning to come back

2 .... All the background noises are coming back again

3 .... I am able to recall the room I'm are in

4 .... I am feeling calm and completely relaxed

5 .... I am aware of my whole body

6 ....I am feeling calm and peaceful

7 .... I am aware of my surroundings and all the
background noises

8 ....Feeling so calm and relaxed

9 .... I begin to open my eyes now

10 .... I open my eyes and come back feeling at peace

Exercise positive statements

- o Everyday I am becoming more fitter and healthier
- o Keeping active makes me strong
- o I love exercising
- o Exercising feels right
- o I exercise everyday and love it
- o I am focussed when working out
- o I always stick to my exercise plan
- o My body is in great shape
- o I feel more healthier with each exercise
- o Exercise comes naturally to me
- o I am in the best shape of my life

- o I let go of my dislike to exercise
- o I am mentally and physically strong
- o Having a healthy body is important to me
- o Exercise allows me to create the body I like
- o I have a strong desire and determination to exercise everyday
- o I am more confident in my abilities and the way I look
- o I let go of being lazy
- o I am highly motivated to stay on track
- o I am proud of myself and my achievements
- o I have good reason to exercise
- o I am reaping the benefits of exercise
- o I look amazing in all my clothes
- o I get a lot of compliments on how good I look
- o I am strong, fit and healthy
- o I enjoy my exercise routine
- o My metabolism speeds up with every workout
- o I am taking full responsibility for my health
- o I have plenty of time to exercise everyday
- o I have taken my power back and I am in control of my well-being

Exercise visualization

Visualizations or mental rehearsal is very popular in sports and physical activity because it boosts confidence, motivation and also primes the body and mind to achieve goals when working out. With plenty of practice mentally creating images will get easier and easier.

Exercise visualization

o Put aside time everyday and practice at least two to three times a day

o Sit in a quiet place and start by breathing in deeply, let go of the tension in your body and close your eyes ....

o Visualize yourself in great detail making that important decision to exercise and, using all your senses, visualize the numerous healthy benefits of exercising.......it will keep you fit, toned and in shape, give you strength, help you lose all the weight you want to lose, reduce stress and relax you, it will boost your confidence and you will sleep better ...... you continue picturing all these healthy benefits and how they will make your life so much better ...... notice how good you feel already ...... and most of all you look good and you're healthy.

o Continue visualizing using all your five senses you imagine yourself starting your exercise or your work out ...... you feel good about yourself and you know that you're going to have a great time ...... you now see yourself exercise ...... you feel so energetic and empowered ...... your mind is focussed and body is responding to your mind ..... they are working in sync .... this feels great and you're actually enjoying it .... you feel in control knowing that you have the power to decide how you look .... and you feel incredible ......

o You now vividly visualize how you want to look like ...... your perfect body and hold on to that mental picture in your mind, see it vividly, how you want to feel and look ...... because you are in the process of creating that ideal body ...... by keeping active everyday ...... in fact the more you exercise the healthier you're and the better you look ...... Visualize a lot of people noticing how good you look ...... and the compliments keep coming in ...... from your family, friends and work colleagues visualize all of them admiring the new you, all healthy, fit and great looking

o Continue to visualize yourself exercising everyday and sticking to your working out plan and it is working out for you perfectly fine ...... you feel and look even better with each day ...... you have more energy, ambition and confidence to carry you on everyday ...... this is an incredible feeling that you want to keep with you ..... you can see and feel first hand that the process is working and it is all happening right now ......

o You continue holding on to that image of a healthier and fitter you, you feel so happy within yourself and fulfilled ...... because you have achieved your goals ...... you exercise everyday and you know that you will continue to do so in the future ...... to make better choices based on your new healthier image ...... You're positive and feel and look good exuding tremendous confidence.

o You believe and trust the process without questioning it because you can feel the transformation already happening within you.

****

Part Six

SELF-MOTIVATION

Motivation is a process or force that pushes us to initiate and maintain goal-directed behaviours or actions. Motivation is powered by desire and any self-motivation should stem from the mind. As mentioned in other chapters, the mind is a very productive tool which, if harnessed in motivation, will yield tremendous benefits whether it is making the right food choices, losing weight or maintaining a healthy weight. Nevertheless, self-motivation will require emotional strength, the ability to be persistent through challenges and also endurance so you keep going matter what hurdles you have to jump. Self-motivation is a quality required for anyone who wants to achieve personal development and success because without it you will give in at the first hurdle and therefore you will have little or no chance in succeeding in whatever you want to achieve.

Motivation will change the way you think about yourself and how you view life as a whole, you will feel more in control of what you want to achieve, when you want to achieve it and how you want to achieve it. Get yourself motivated, stay motivated and your dreams will become a reality! Whatever it is that you're aiming to achieve whether it is losing weight, managing your weight, keeping active or sticking to a healthy eating plan, motivation is guaranteed to help you go that extra mile.

Motivation has major stages which are;

1- **Activation-** this is the first step when you make that decision to initiate action and bring about the desired changes.

2- **Persistence-** Is the continuity and perseverance with the actions to change a behaviour or attain a goal. You will have to oversee all the difficulties that arise and keep focussed to achieve your goal. This will also require your time, energy and resources.

3- **Intensity-** This is a certain degree of power and energy that you will need to sustain you through your self-motivation process.

Self Hypnosis for motivation

Self-hypnosis for motivation helps with getting rid of any past negative programming, improving self-projection, increasing confidence, self-acceptance and changing your perspective on how you deal with problems or challenges.

MOTIVATION SCRIPT

I will make myself as comfortable as I can ...... take a deep breath ...... close my eyes and begin to relax ...... and allow myself to let go ...... just thinking about relaxing every muscle in my body ..... from the top of my head to the tips of my toes ...... as I begin to focus attention on my breathing ...... my awareness of everything around me will decrease ...... and as I continue to do this I can feel all the tension and stress leave my mind and body ....

I begin to drift into a deeper and deeper relaxation ...... feeling lighter and lighter ...... I let go of everything completely .... relaxing even more ..... now that I am completely relaxed ...... more relaxed than I have ever felt before ...... and as I experience this beautiful feeling of peace and calm ...... I am going to allow myself to work with my subconscious mind to accept all the suggestions .... without being critical of them .... and analysing them ...... I will follow them and I will be more motivated than ever to accomplish my goals ......

Now that I am deeply relaxed and ready to take in and accept all the suggestions .... I am imagining myself in my special place ...... I can feel it and see it .... this is the most peaceful place in the world for me .... here I am alone and there is no one to disturb me or ask for anything .... its just me ...... in my special place .... my special time .... I can feel a sense of peace flow through me .... and a sense of well-being .... as I continue to relax deeper and deeper .... Because I am deeply relaxed now .... my subconscious mind will accept the new suggestions .... because it hears everything and always pays attention ...... and strives to work towards my well-being ...... for my motivation and self empowerment .... I will reach all my goals and become a successful person with nothing holding me back .... from this very moment starting right now I will push back all the barriers that I have created in the past .... and instead I am creating opportunities and expanding my horizons .... achieving my goals ...... reaching higher and higher with each day .... feeling comfortable and at ease with my expanded boundaries .... and sticking to them easily ...... I eat a healthy balanced meal everyday because being healthy is my main priority ...... I feel secure and pleased that I have control and power within myself to stick to my new healthy eating plan .... to change my limitations and be the successful person I want to be ...... the person I deserve to be ...... and I feel good ...... confident ...... at peace and content with my choices ...... now I imagine myself exercising everyday .... getting even more healthier and fitter ...... and it feels just fine because I am motivated more than ever before to stick to my workout routine ...... and it works perfectly fine for me ...... because I am in total control of myself and my well-being and taking all the precautions to eat healthier .... exercise daily and attain my goal weight .... taking charge with a positive mind set ..... right now ....

I am now free of past burdens ..... I am secure .... confident .... self-assured and I feel centred and strong ..... now I am imagining all the goals I want to achieve .... I see new opportunities and new challenges that are more exciting than the old ones .... I see myself with renewed energy ..... I am enthusiastic and focussed than ever before .... new ideas develop and positive feelings ...... I am reaching for my goal ...... I am successful and I am worthy of all the good things life has to offer ...... reaching my goals is very beneficial to me ...... and as I continue to reach the goals in my life ...... with a positive frame of mind ..... I will embrace all positive opportunities coming up for me .... I reflect on all the other things I have achieved in my life .... and know that I am capable of succeeding again .... in reaching my all goals ...... I see myself become successful ...... I am happy and comfortable in my success .... I use my success in positive and worthwhile ways ...... I deserve to be healthy and fit it's my right ...... I can see it ...... I can feel it ...... because it is happening right now ..... starting from today ...... I see myself as healthy, fit, strong and confident ...... I have many choices and options .... and whatever direction I choose to take .... I know it will be the right one for me ...... every choice and direction I take from now on will be the absolute right one for me ...... I can see myself clearly in the future with many positive and healthy choices for me ...... and I bring this image to the present ...... and I see myself choosing the healthy options again and again .... because its the only proven and tested choice that works for me ...... I am confident with my perfect choice ..... and I know I will continue to be successful and it will work out for me to positively enhance my life ...... I remain in this relaxed and peaceful state for a few more minutes to enjoy these wonderful feelings ...... enjoying being here in my special place knowing that I can always come back here whenever I wish to experience these positive feeling again and again .... and bring them back with me to the present ..... drifting and floating ...... relaxing ....

In a few minutes I will come back to awareness .... I will count from one to ten and as I count from one to ten......I will begin to come back to full awareness ...... calm and relaxed.

1 ....Beginning to come back

2 ....The background noises are coming back

3 ....Feeling relaxed

4 ....I am starting to recall the room I am in

5 ....Feeling completely calm and relaxed

6 ....I am aware of my whole body

7 .... Feeling very peaceful

8 .... I am aware of my surroundings and all the background noises

9 ....I begin to open my eyes

10 ....I open my eyes and come back feeling at peace and relaxed

Self-motivation positive statements

- o I am more motivated than ever before to achieve my goals
- o I am a highly motivated and determined person
- o I am motivated at all times
- o I am always motivated and always get things done on time
- o I am motivated to eat a balanced meal everyday
- o I find it easy to motivate myself to enhance my well-being
- o I am motivated to stay healthy and fit
- o My positive energy motivates me to achieve my goals
- o I am becoming more and more motivated every single day
- o I find motivation within myself other than from other people
- o I am my own motivator and make my dreams into a reality

o I am getting more and more driven and ambitious
o I am hugely motivated and productive
o I am becoming more and more motivated to exercise
o Each day I wake up more motivated to be active
o Being motivated is part of who I am
o Being motivated drives me to achieve success
o Motivation comes naturally for me
o I can do anything I set my mind to
o Motivation helps me maintain a healthy weight
o I release all negativity in my life and only focus on positive aspects of life
o I keep a positive frame of mind and positive things happen in my life
o I take on challenges and view them as opportunities to grow
o Motivation comes to me from inside.
o I am my own motivator when it comes to losing weight
o With motivation I can achieve anything
o I deserve the best out of life because I am a worthy human being
o I always give my best and reap good rewards
o I am successful through motivation
o Motivation leads the way to success

Self-help tips for motivation

o Set yourself goals which are realistic and achievable, this will make it easier for you to motivate yourself to move forward to where you want to be.

o Be persistent and patient, however much work your goal is to achieve, don't give up just because you've had a set back, see challenges as opportunities for you to learn, grow and move on. Success is all about grafting.

o Positive thinking will take you a long way so keep positive and try and eliminate negativity out of life. Focus on the good things rather than the bad.

o Set yourself a deadline and stick with it, when you have achieved your goal reward yourself for the hard work.

o Socialise with people who inspire you and keep you motivated.

o Visualization techniques will help you create a mental picture of what you want to achieve. Seeing yourself already achieving your goal makes your brain believe that attaining that goal is possible. Focussing consistently on your goal will enable you to manifest it sooner and bring it within your grasp.

****

Index

****

Other Publications In This Series

SELF-HYPNOSIS AND POSITIVE AFFIRMATIONS
THE ART OF SELF
THERAPY

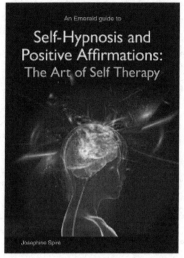

Hypnosis is the gentle healer, no chemicals, no side effects and it puts the patient in a state that holds great potential for healing by giving the patient access to the subconscious mind.

Self- Hypnosis and Positive Affirmations-The Art of Self Therapy is a book about how hypnosis combined with positive affirmations can be powerful in treating a number of physical, psychological, stress related disorders, phobias and promoting sporting performance among others. This book is original and practical and will benefit anyone who wishes to investigate further. More and more people are beginning to realise and appreciate the healing power of hypnosis and affirmations

ISBN: 978-1-84716-499-5 Price: £9.99

143